The Secret of Health:
BREAST WISDOM

BEN JOHNSON
AND
KATHLEEN BARNES

New York

The Secret of Health: Breast Wisdom

Library of Congress Number: 2007938782
ISBN: 978-1-60037-326-8 (Paperback)
ISBN: 978-1-60037-327-5 (Hardcover)

Published by:

MORGAN · JAMES
THE ENTREPRENEURIAL PUBLISHER
www.morganjamespublishing.com

Morgan James Publishing, LLC
1225 Franklin Ave. Ste 325
Garden City, NY 11530-1693
Toll Free 800-485-4943
www.MorganJamesPublishing.com

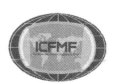

International Cancer Foundation Management Foundation is a non-profit organization dedicated to researching natural cures for cancer and providing for those who cannot afford them. The Foundation is also engaged in many other Christian activities.

Cover Design by:
Cathi Stevenson
www.bookcoverexpress.com

Interior Design by:
Sabra Hammond
sabrahammond@yahoo.com

DEDICATION FROM DR. BEN:

For Jill Jarrett:

It is because of her that this book was written. In hope that no woman armed with the knowledge within should ever have to go through what she went through. And for those she left behind: Jeff, Joslyn, Jaclyn and Jeryn. I love all of you. Jill, I will see you on the other side.

And for Sharon Dubreuil:

To the girl who saw her mother die of breast cancer, lived with the fear and overcame it. I honor you and those women who have the courage to rise above the fear.

ACKNOWLEDGEMENTS

For all those who brought their patience, diligence and dedication to the creation of this book, we are deeply grateful.

We are especially grateful for the contributions of Dr. Ben's capable and brilliant assistant, Kimberly Johnson, whose organizational skills and proofreading abilities were invaluable.

And to Cathi Stevenson for her beautiful design and Sabra Hammond for her eye catching graphic design, we thank you.

Last, but not least, we extend our gratitude to our families for their forbearance during interrupted family outings and delayed family time and for their love and support during the process of birthing this book.

FROM DR. BEN: I extend special thanks to my children who gave up so many hours with their dad that they love so much and most of all for my beautiful, incredible wife who gave the most to see me through this adventure in my life. You are the best !

FROM BOTH OF US: To our families: We love you. You are a blessing in our lives.

— *Dr. Ben Johnson and Kathleen Barnes*

TABLE OF CONTENTS

FOREWORD

When I was sixteen, as I was showering and getting ready for the day, I noticed my breast felt harder. Immediately a wave of fear rushed through me. Like every young girl, I had heard the horror stories about breast cancer. I was scared to death. Night after sleepless night, I laid in bed worrying about what to do. Should I tell my mom, should I talk to my big sister, should I go see the nurse at school? As it turned out, there was nothing wrong. But the panic and fear I experienced is the same fear experienced by millions of girls and women throughout the world everyday. The lack of knowledge and education about healthy and effective means of preventing and treating breast cancer is what has been missing. I wish this book was available for my mother to have read to me when I was younger.

Kudos to Dr. Ben Johnson and Kathleen Barnes. Finally, a book that covers absolutely everything a woman needs to know about the prevention and maintenance of healthy breasts! Leaving no stone unturned, "Breast Wisdom" is an easy to read, down to earth book that is both thought provoking and knowledge packed. Beginning with the first stages of a woman's breast to menopause, "Breast Wisdom" educates women about the many different cycles, changes and concerns she needs to be aware of in order to have a healthy relationship with her breasts.

With chapters educating women about the type of nutrients she needs, to the various techniques she can practice daily for clarity of mind, and the specific exercises that she can do on a daily basis to keep her body in top physical condition, this book never fails to bring to light knowledge that uplifts and educates. One of the most unique features of this book is that it shows a woman how to integrate the most advanced scientific knowledge about energetic healing techniques with other alternative and traditional healing modalities step-by-step. On top of that, it also dares to cover the controversial side effects of the treatments and drugs that the medical profession routinely prescribes to women with breast cancer. It is my hope that this book will be made mandatory to educate young girls all over the world about one of the most important issues they will ever face.

 —*Janet Bray Attwood,*
  bestselling author,
  The Passion Test -
  The Effortless Path to Discovering Your Destiny

INTRODUCTION

This is a book about health. It's not surprising that most of us don't pay much attention to our bodies until something goes wrong, so it's also not surprising that many women don't think much about breast health unless something goes wrong.

There are lots of books on the market that say they are about breast health, but they are really about breast cancer. This isn't a book about breast cancer. It's a book about breast health.

In this book, we'll address myriad ways to keep your breasts healthy. Of course we'll talk about breast cancer, prevention and what to do if you get it, because it is a big concern for so many women. Yet our major focus is on health in all its many aspects. We'll show you ways to recover your health if something goes wrong.

We think we've created a good team for this book.

Dr. Ben has the expertise as an integrative oncologist, highly trained and deeply experienced in helping women keep their breasts healthy and helping women regain breast health if they have had cancer.

And Kathleen is a deeply experienced journalist, author of six books, five on natural health and editor of several more. In addition, Kathleen is deeply committed to natural healing. She also brings to this book her experience as a woman.

Early in the writing process, we considered calling this book Breasts: An Owner's Manual. That seemed a lot like a car manual, and we quickly discarded the idea. The subject has evolved since then, largely because of Dr. Ben's involvement with *The Healing Codes*™ and his appearance in *The Secret*™. Both of us are firm believers in the power of the mind and emotions to create change in our physical bodies, our families and our world. We also understand that the process of health, specifically breast health, is far more than physical. That is the breast wisdom we share with you.

Our focus is on the positive. You get what you think about. Think about health.

We'd like to share with you a bit of our stories here:

DR. BEN SAYS: It has been my personal honor to stand by the sides of many women when something goes wrong, terribly wrong, and they must combat the ravages of disease. I hope I have offered some comfort and I know I have offered healing to many in unconventional ways.

I'm there to help them make the right choices when hard choices are presented, to fight their way back to health, and yes, sometimes to die, since death is indeed life's final adventure for every single one of us on this earth.

I've had my experience with illness and I know what it means to create the health and vital life all of us want.

Let's go back to September of 2002. I was living in Georgia with my wonderful wife and seven awesome children.

I had an alternative medical clinic which was going along very well. I felt I was helping many people who were not being helped by conventional medicine, and it was immensely fulfilling.

Then I began to get some little muscle twitches called fasciculations. As a doctor, I knew what they were; I just didn't know why my muscles in particular were choosing to do this at this time.

I made the mistake of ignoring them, thinking they were related to a spinal cord injury I had a few years earlier.

The problem worsened until it looked like I had worms crawling under my skin. I got so weak I could hardly walk up a flight of stairs. My voice got weak.

Finally, I went to see an orthopedic surgeon. He told me I had Lou Gehrig's disease, amyotrophic lateral sclerosis, a degenerative disease of the motor nerves that almost inevitably leads to death. I didn't like the diagnosis—who would? But I faced the reality when a second doctor confirmed the diagnosis.

It took me exactly a fraction of a millisecond to realize I was in big trouble. I knew that conventional medicine had absolutely nothing to offer. I even knew that the doctor who had an office next door to mine was doing some research on stem cell transplants for patients with ALS, but then the government shut down the study because it showed no long-term benefit.

And I was the alternative medicine doctor. I had tried to help ALS patients with herbs, nutritionals, homeopathics, energy, frequency devices and acupunture. Frankly, nothing I had tried had helped.

I started looking for life insurance policies worth a couple of million dollars, praying I could stay alive for at least two years so my wife and seven children could collect the insurance and be in good shape financially. I'm not proud of that, but that's the way it was.

There was absolutely nothing I could do about this disease.

My life changed dramatically in February 2003 when I met Alex Loyd, the creator of *The Healing Codes*™, a system that uses quantum physics to help heal cells damaged by trauma that he believes (and I confirm!) are the cause of almost all illness.

A light came on for me. I'd never seen anything like that, but, as a scientist, it made sense to me.

Without delay, I began applying *The Healing Codes*™. Within six weeks, I began to get noticeable improvement in my physical symptoms. Within eight weeks, I was confident I had reversed the disease process.

Today, nearly five years later, when 80 percent of the people with Lou Gehrig's disease would already be dead, not only am I alive and kicking, I am healthy and vital.

Every once in a while, I get a little muscle jiggle under my skin, and I take that as a reminder that the potential for the disease is still there for me if I don't stay emotionally clear and live in love. That's what I believe and my life is centered around that belief.

It's that experience that has sparked my passion to share the route to natural healing with as many people as possible.

My family is glad I'm still around—and so am I. This second lease on life gives me an opportunity to share some insights into healing that are life-changing for everyone.

KATHLEEN SAYS: I think I've always known the secrets of the Law of Attraction, but, like everyone, I tend to forget how profoundly my thought processes affect my world.

When Dr. Ben first called me on one snowy Saturday night in February, my husband and I were watching a video of *The Secret*™. I was somewhat annoyed to be interrupted, but, being a mom, I picked up the phone in case my daughter needed me. I wasn't prepared to get a business call from an unknown doctor at 11 p.m. on a Saturday, nor was I prepared for the ways that call would change my life. That first conversation was very short since I rather sternly informed Dr. Ben that we were having "family time."

When we connected during normal business hours a couple of days later, Dr. Ben asked how our "family time" had been.

"It was good," I told him. "We were watching a movie called *The Secret*™. Have you heard of it?"

There was a pregnant few seconds of silence.

Then he quietly replied, "Yes. I'm in it."

After I recovered from the rush of adrenaline of learning about the Law of Attraction in such an "out there" manner, I knew this was a book that I had to write.

Since my early twenties, I've had a passion for natural healing. Of course, back in those days, alternative medicine was considered extremely fringe and "free radicals" were probably related to political extremists, not natural healing.

I began teaching yoga and practicing meditation and living a natural lifestyle. It served me well over the ensuing decades.

Now, a few years down the road and six natural health books under my belt, I know I have found a way to express my true passion, and like Dr. Ben, I can share with readers what I've learned along the way.

As the owner of a healthy pair of breasts, I have learned an immense amount in working with Dr. Ben and in researching this book. What I thought I knew sometimes turned out not to be true and what I didn't know was vast. I'm thankful for the opportunity to learn more every day. And I'm still not wearing my bra most of the time! (See Chapter 3 for an explanation.)

—*Ben Johnson, M.D., D.O., N.M.D.*
Rossville, Georgia
—*Kathleen Barnes*
Brevard, North Carolina
May 2007

Chapter 1 THE AMERICAN LOVE AFFAIR WITH BREASTS

From the time a girl reaches the tender age of eight or so, she starts to think about her breasts. She may touch her flat breast, push up imaginary cleavage and model in front of the mirror in eager anticipation of the day those magical mammaries will appear.

When she becomes a teenager, she actually has breasts. These newfound appendages are the object of much fascination, and not just for the boys who so delight in watching them emerge. Not only do breasts warrant mirror time, teenage girls spend a great deal of time looking down at their chests, perhaps to confirm the continuing presence of these wondrous objects.

As a young woman matures, her breasts become a source of pleasure and delight for herself and her husband.

Then comes motherhood and those beautiful breasts become the source of life for our babies. Those still, small moments shared by a mother and her baby as Mom rocks and Baby suckles are among the most intimate ones a woman will ever know.

A few years later in life, as gravity begins to have its way with all human tissue, we begin to worry. Are they drooping? Should I have implants to shore things up? Some saline support? And the one we don't even want to give voice to: What is that lump?

As she gets older and the risks increase, she may become preoccupied with the fear of losing a breast. Some women actually refuse to be examined for fear of a diagnosis that would cause them to be disfigured or lose a breast altogether.

This book is not primarily about breast cancer. It's about healthy breasts, happy breasts and keeping your breasts both happy and healthy.

Yes, we will talk about breast cancer, much later in this book, after you've learned what a healthy breast looks and feels like and what you need to do to keep your breasts that way.

The secrets of *The Secret*™

It's important to start with an understanding of a basic law of the universe on which we approach our lives and, for purposes of this book, our health: Your thought processes are reflected in your body and in the world around you. If you constantly worry that you aren't good enough, you never will be good enough until you change your way of thinking.

Many of you have probably seen Rhonda Byrne's remarkable film, *The Secret*™ or read her book by the same title. If you haven't, we recommend that you see the film. Dr. Ben is in both the film and the book.

We'll give you a quick synopsis here:

The secret is the Law of Attraction. What does that mean? The message the other teachers and Dr. Ben brought to you in the *The Secret* ™ is that your state of mind influences your world. It means your feelings and thoughts attract real events into your life to some degree. What you think about yourself and your world helps to influence what your world becomes.

Did you ever notice how certain people seem to have a magic touch? Think of someone you know who did well in school, won all the awards, has the best job, the right mate and lives a healthy and fulfilling life.

Now think of someone you know whose life is a daily struggle. These are the folks who walk down the street looking at the pavement, who time after time wind up in destructive relationships, are always on the brink of financial disaster and are beset with a wide array of health problems.

The difference between these two types of people is how they think of themselves and their lives.

The people who live abundant, fulfilling lives are almost without exception those who have a strong positive self-image and who see the world as their oyster. Those with continuing challenges almost always engage in a stream of negative self-talk in which they see themselves as stupid, lazy, unlucky or useless. That negative self-image creates a life of poverty, illness, loneliness and fear.

Who wants it? Breaking those lifelong thought patterns is a challenge, but any of us can change our lives by changing the way we think of ourselves and our world and feeling how those new thought patterns create an energetic shift in ourselves and finally, to act on those new patterns.

It's really as simple as that.

DR. BEN SAYS: The Law of Attraction is a real phenomenon. It exists, and works in real time. We need to be using it in a positive fashion. We also need to be careful about misusing this principle. So where should our focus be? Well let's examine where these principles came from and work from there.

The Law of Attraction is found in ancient manuscripts such as the Bible and in other places. The Bible says, "For whatsoever a person sows, that is what they will reap," and "As a person thinks in their heart so are they."

There are also encouragements to always be thankful and to have a thankful heart.

There are other texts that we should not forget in this context: "It is in giving that we receive" and "It is better to give than to receive."

However there is a greater principle than all of these. When He was asked, "What is the most important thing of all, Jesus replied, "Love."

We need to be careful not to make the Law of Attraction an exercise in getting "stuff" for ourselves. Cars, houses, the boat, and the plane – these can be good things. They can also be a wrong goal if it's about getting stuff for ourselves instead of giving.

I think we would do well to make the focus of our attraction about giving, about living in love, being in integrity and paying ahead.

In case some of us don't know what paying ahead is, it is doing something for someone who can't give back to you. It's about a way of life that is centered around living life out of love.

In a few years, the expensive car will be in a junk yard, plastic rotted by the sun, glass broken, metal rusting. The fashion outfit that we bought – well it's already out of style. You see stuff is just stuff. It has no eternal value.

The only thing that matters is others and living in love, light and integrity with those around us. That is how we can best use the Law of Attraction.

More secrets from *The Healing Codes*™

Now let's take *The Secret*™ a step further. In my work with Dr. Alexander Loyd, we've found *The Healing Codes*™, a simple system that can bring about healing of deep-seated memories that are stored in our cells. We believe the heart is the seat of our unconscious and subconscious mind. Science calls this cellular memory.

These cellular memories contain wrong beliefs about ourselves, others, life and God. These beliefs create physiological stress. With enough stress over time, something physical is often the first thing to give, usually resulting in health problems.

The Healing Codes™ are a physical mechanism built into the human body that consistently and predictably removes stress from the body. *The Healing Codes*™ activate what appears to work like a hidden fuse box. Stress breaks the circuit. The codes flip the correct circuits open, allowing the healing of almost any illness.

We believe, and we have support from Dr. Bruce Lipton, a Stanford biologist who may have been the first person to identify spiritual heart issues from a scientific perspective, that if you heal the cellular memory that causes stress, illness and disease can heal as well.

To give just one example that is really pertinent to many women: If you believe that you are not worthy of love, you are believing a lie and denying the truth of who you really are. By re-connecting the circuit and ending that belief in a very simple way, the stress (or the lie) is removed and you are healed. Then you can live life from a different place.

We'll be giving you much more detail about *The Healing Codes*™ in Chapter 5. For now, just keep these concepts in your mind: If you hold limiting beliefs, you are not basking in the perfect physical, emotional and spiritual health that is everyone's birthright. Using some simple tools to change those beliefs will bring about healing on all levels.

Thinking of your breasts in a different way

DR. BEN SAYS: I think women in general continuously ask themselves, "Am I good enough?" This absolutely includes their breasts. This deep seated fear of inadequacy is rooted among 21st century women who juggle home, family, work and volunteerism. It would be a laughing matter if it weren't so serious. It's wrecking women's health.

So we can take the lessons of the Law of Attraction and apply them to our way of thinking about our breasts.

If you're constantly worrying about whether they're big enough or firm enough or whether you might get cancer, you're creating energetic patterns that directly affect your health.

I have noticed in my practice that those who fear cancer the most have a greater risk of getting cancer. Their minds are continually chanting a Fear of Cancer mantra and so, thinking about the Law of Attraction, you can imagine what they often receive.

Imagine what it would be like if all women thought of their breasts as whole, healthy and perfect just as they are. Imagine, even more importantly, that we could heal the feelings of anger, fear, frustration and pain and re-set our cellular memories to messages of health and wholeness. I think the rate of breast cancer would decrease dramatically.

That's exactly what we are presenting to you here.

Body image

Today's society has given us some pretty quirky notions about the ideal woman: She should be tall, slender as a reed with long legs, tiny taut hips, a perfect complexion, long wavy naturally blond hair and, of course, perfect, high, plump breasts.

In other words, she should look exactly like Barbie. Did you know that the Barbie doll's absurd and unnatural proportions would force her to crawl on all fours if she were human? Yet this is the image of perfect womanhood we have presented to our young girls for two generations now. Or at least it used to be that way. Now we like big booties, as well as breasts.

We're here to tell you that Barbie doesn't represent the norm at all. Neither do supermodels.

Kathleen finds this unattainable and undesirable body image to be particularly upsetting since it has led to eating disorders and poor self-esteem for generations of girls.

DR. BEN SAYS: In my years of practice, I've performed 10,000 pelvic and breast exams. That's 20,000 breasts. I can count on my fingers and toes the ones who look like the models in the magazines. Truthfully, even the models don't look like that. They're airbrushed. There are three billion women in the world and eight of them look like supermodels. The supermodels are the ones who are abnormal. The images in magazines and the media are not normal. Think of the Law of Attraction and how these images impact the self-image of women who don't look like that.

Most of our readers are women and most of you understand the emotional link women have to their breasts.

It's difficult to explain that deep sense of self-identity connected with breasts that goes far beyond the simple physical function they serve to nourish our babies.

Breasts are an external manifestation of womanhood. A woman can lose an appendix, a gall bladder, even a uterus and, while the loss of an organ may be upsetting, it can't compare to the deep grief that many women feel if they are even asked to consider the idea that they might lose a breast.

KATHLEEN SAYS: *Breasts are the ultimate manifestation of ourselves as women. I know this is not entirely logical, since a woman is perfectly capable of conceiving and delivering a healthy child in the absence of breasts. So who ever said the world is logical? We all know in our minds that it is the uterus, not the breast that is the vessel for the ultimate feminine power to bring new life into this world. And, yes, women who lose their uteruses for whatever reason often grieve, but the loss of the uterus is nothing like the loss of self-identity that accompanies the loss or surgical disfigurement of a breast. Maybe it's simply that the psychic wound is re-opened every day through the brutal honesty of the mirror.*

I honor those she-roes who proudly display their post-mastectomy flattened chests, festoon them with tattoos and hold their heads high. Yet I know these women are few and far between. Most women who have suffered this loss suffer in silence. My heart goes out to them.

Breasts have a unique place in the American culture. They're a matter of national obsession. Yes, of course, they are a strangely paradoxical sex object. We'll explain what we mean by that in a few paragraphs, but bear with us: For both men and women, breasts are icons of sexuality.

Our advertising, our movies, our fashions and even our body language emphasize this fascination with the glories of the female breast. How many times have you seen teenage girls preen themselves in their tight-fitting t-shirts while teenage boys ogle them?

These things are a normal part of life, you might say. Well, they maybe in America, but not so in other parts of the world.

In Africa and parts of Asia, breasts are not sex objects. Most tribal women do not wear bras. Often they don't even wear any garments that cover their breasts. In those areas, breasts are simply parts of the body that feed babies. True, women's breasts sag and gravity eventually takes its toll. They are not sexual and no one gives them a second thought.

Even the westernized Europeans are nowhere nearly as obsessed with breasts as are Americans. We've made an art of it!

Ironically, most breastfeeding women reveal far less skin than the average Victoria's Secret commercial reveals. Yet many people find one inappropriate and the other attractive.

We Americans have a paradoxical phobia about breasts when they are used for the purpose for which they were intended: feeding babies. Many people get squeamish when a woman breast feeds her baby in public. Some municipalities have actually banned public breastfeeding and required nursing mothers to take their babies into public bathrooms to feed them. Bathrooms are hardly sanitary places for babies or comfortable places for nursing!

A local regulation comes to mind that involved a group of women who were told they could not breast feed their babies at a community swimming pool. That seemed especially absurd since the bathing suits many women wear today cover far less than a baby's head would cover while it is nursing. The swimming pool moms and many others are quite rightly fighting these local regulations.

Breast augmentation, is it for you?

We want to clearly state that we are not judging or condemning any woman who has or may get breast augmentation. However, we feel compelled to share that it is not always an upside, that there are downsides too. Nevertheless, we completely understand why many women choose to have plastic surgery on their breasts. After all, isn't that what makeup is about, looking nice? Every woman wants to feel beautiful!

Dr. Ben has a niece, who, after four children, had inverted nipples. She was so self-conscious of her breasts and even more concerned about how she looked to her husband that she could think of nothing else. So breast augmentation is OK. It can be a very good thing bringing joy, happiness and an increase in your sense of femininity. Just be aware of all the possibilities before you make your choice.

The good news is there is no increase in breast cancer associated with implants. Implants do make it more difficult for you and your doctor to effectively examine your breasts, so you'll both have to take special care.

The density of the implants can block the ability of mammograms to look into questionable areas, but we don't recommend mammograms anyway, in most cases. (See Chapter 5) That's one of many reasons why we recommend yearly thermograms.

Breast implants are a major surgical procedure that can have significant consequences. We say that because this surgery carries all of the risks of any other surgery: General anesthesia, infection, rejection and disfigurement. Yet 12 million women choose this surgical procedure every year, most of them paying the cost out of their own pockets. There are even doctors who will finance the breast implant surgery for "only $99 down and payments."

In addition to the risks anyone takes with surgery and general anesthesia, some women who have breast enlargements have experienced extreme nipple sensitivity or sometimes complete numbness, scar tissue that causes the breast to become hard and infection that requires additional surgery.

What ever you do, if you do choose augmentation, do it for you, not for someone else. Do not look for a quick fix of an emotional issue with a cosmetic surgical procedure.

DR. BEN SAYS: There is also an emotional risk involved in breast augmentation. I am not sure I can completely explain how this happens, but it changes a woman's view of her breasts including how modest she is. For example, I clearly remember the first physical exam I performed on an implant patient. I read over her history and when I asked about her implant surgery, she cheerfully pulled up her blouse and showed her new breasts to me. They were indeed impressive, but the point is that I have never had any other woman in my entire medical career so willingly show her breasts. Somehow her breasts had become something to show off, rather than something personal and private.

In conclusion

Breasts are indeed a part of the female anatomy that should be celebrated, acknowledged and appreciated. Over the next few days, spend some time giving serious consideration to your way of thinking about your breasts. They are beautiful; they are you. We want you to know how best to care for them and keep them.

Chapter 2

WHAT DO HEALTHY BREASTS LOOK AND FEEL LIKE?

Breasts come in an endless variety of sizes and shapes. Some are very dense and firm to the touch. Others are quite large, light and compressible, what we'd call "fluffy."

They can feel bumpy; they may be noticeably different in size. Nipples may be large, very dark colored no matter what the skin tone or they might be very pale colored. Nipples may be permanently erect or small, light pink and flat unless aroused.

The only benchmark we can give you is to tell you that there isn't a benchmark. Just about "anything goes" when it comes to how breasts look and feel. What is normal is what you have – at least it's normal for you.

Since our culture generally doesn't give women permission to be bare breasted, even with other women, many women really have no grounds for comparison, unless they take a few quick peeks at the men's magazines. Don't go there! Those women are not real. They are airbrushed, specially lighted and even computer enhanced. Heaven knows what other tactics are used to make them look that way. Don't expect you'll look like them. Nobody does, not even the models themselves.

The lack of information can lead to fear and speculation that something is wrong when in fact, everything is quite normal.

This chapter is going to give you the true picture of the anatomy of breasts, how they develop, the way breasts function at various times of a woman's life, breast self-examination and when you should and should not get worried.

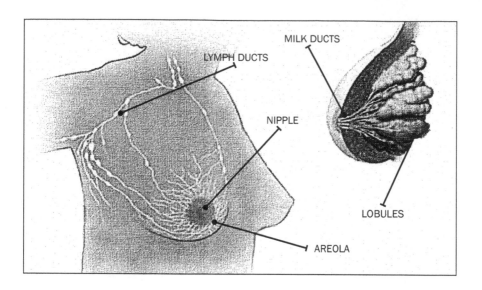

MILK DUCTS

LYMPH DUCTS

NIPPLE

LOBULES

AREOLA

The anatomy of a breast

Of course, both men and women have breasts, but men's breasts have little physiological function.

The bulk of breast tissue is fat and fibrous connective tissue that binds the breast together and gives it shape. Inside the female breast are 15 to 25 milk-producing sacs called milk glands. These milk glands come together inside the nipple.

On the outside of the breast is the nipple and the surrounding circular areola, an extension of the skin of the nipple containing many nerve fibers that help the nipple to stiffen and become erect.

What should a normal female breast look like?

There's no such thing as a "normal" breast. Every single one is different, so please erase from your consciousness the question of whether your breasts are "normal" or not. Look in the mirror: What you see is normal. Really! What is important and what we hope to impress upon you is that every woman should know her breasts intimately. Size, shape, color – none of these are important. What is important is knowing the normal configurations of your own breasts and then when you are very familiar with them you will know if anything changes.

One of the concerns that women most often express to Dr. Ben is the lack of symmetry in their breasts. Breasts of unequal size are common. In fact, perfectly symmetrical breasts are rare. Often, the left breast is larger because of the way the arteries run from the aorta, providing a slightly better blood supply to the left breast and sometimes making it grow larger. But that's a rule that's made to be broken, so don't get worried if your right breast is larger than your left.

Usually the difference isn't terribly noticeable, but it can be. Dr. Ben couldn't help but notice on a recent trip to the optician that the lady adjusting his glasses was probably a D cup on the right side and an EEEE on the left. This dramatic difference might be a little unsettling if you are the one trying to find a bra that fits. However, in and of itself, having breasts of different sizes is not a sign of trouble at all and falls well within the mainstream.

Not only can the breasts be different sizes, they can even be different shapes. This should also be no cause for concern as long as they have always been that way.

Breast shape and appearance undergo a number of changes as a woman ages. In young women, the breast skin stretches and expands as the breasts grow, creating a rounded appearance. Young women tend to have denser breasts (more glandular tissue) than older women. As women age, the ligaments supporting the breasts become weakened and they sag – a bit or a lot.

Nipples also come in all sizes and shapes. In some women, the nipples are permanently erect and very prominent. In others, nipples are flattened unless they are responding to cold or touch. Nipples may be set deep in the breast or even inverted. Inverted nipples are cause for concern only if they are a sudden development rather than the usual state of affairs. A nipple can be flat, round, or oblong in shape.

Nipples can be very dark colored, regardless of the woman's skin tone, or they can be light and pale pink. There are hair follicles around the nipple, so hair on the breast is not uncommon.

The size and color of the areola is equally variable. Some women have small pink ones and others have larger darker colored ones or vice-versa. Remember, there is no hard and fast definition about what is normal or even average. Many women have small bumps in the areola. These are oil-producing glands that produce a lubricant that helps make breast-feeding easier. When a woman gets pregnant, the areolae darken in color and most often they stay dark after she gives birth.

What determines breast size?

Many women ask Dr. Ben how they can make their breasts larger. The answer to that one is: You can't. Let us qualify that a little. Your breast size may increase if you do certain types of muscle enhancing exercise, since there is a muscle layer underneath the fatty and fibrous

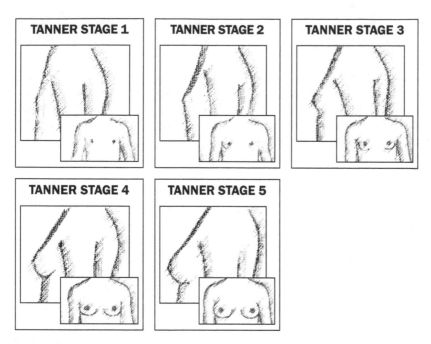

breast tissue. Yes, that old exercise chant, "I must, I must, I must improve my bust," actually has some basis in fact. If you strengthen the underlying muscles, your breasts will become slightly larger, but not much. If you stop exercising this muscle, they will return to their previous size.

However, as we know, exercise burns fat and the breasts are mainly fatty tissue, so with increased exercise, you will end up with more muscle and less fat in the breast tissue. In the end, there will probably be little difference in size, but you may notice a bit more firmness.

Other factors that can affect breast size:

- Family history
- Age
- Weight loss or gain
- History of pregnancies and breast feeding
- Thickness and elasticity of the breast skin — if you have fair skin, you most likely have "thin skin"
- Degree of hormonal influences on the breast (particularly estrogen and progesterone). Breasts often become larger at certain stages of the menstrual cycle and typically shrink slightly after your period. Taking birth control pills or hormone replacement therapy can also cause some changes in breast size.
- Menopause

When a girl becomes a woman

As girls mature, their breasts and other secondary sexual characteristics (including development of pubic hair) follow a series of fairly predictable stages.

The Tanner Staging system, also called the sexual maturity rating, is based on 20 years of research on young girls and their transition through puberty by a British pediatrician, James Tanner, M.D. The five-stage process details exactly what is happening at any given time in a girl's development and predicts with a great deal of accuracy when she will reach menarche or the beginning of her menstrual period.

- *Stage one:* The breast shows no outwardly noticeable changes.

- *Stage two:* Also known as thelarche (the beginning of breast development at puberty), the breast has an areola, the small darkened area around the nipple, the papillary (nipple) mound that may be visible, and a breast bud that can be identified by touch. Tanner found the average age of thelarche was 11.15 years, with a range of 8.5 to 13 years, but that was 40 years ago. These days, girls are maturing much earlier, probably because of xenoestrogens, hormones in our food and in the plastics that are ever present in our society. We'll talk more about that a little later. Another possible cause is visual input from our society and TV related to sexuality. These days, pediatricians don't get too upset if a girl reaches thelarche or Tanner Stage 2 at the age of 8. Still, it's more common today for a girl to start breast development at about age 10.

- *Stage three:* The breast buds are enlarging beyond the edges of the areola. There may be some difference in color between the areola and the other breast tissue that is beginning to grow, but the mound is an even curve without the puckering and differentiation of the areola from the breast that we usually see in mature women. Tanner found that the average age for this stage was 12.15 years, but we can probably subtract at least a year for modern-day girls. African-American girls often mature much earlier and their average ages at these stages can easily be a year or more earlier than 21st century Caucasian girls. Recent studies show African–American girls often reach Stage 3 shortly after their tenth birthdays.

- *Stage four:* This stage may happen very quickly or not at all. Some girls jump directly to Stage 5 without really entering Stage 4. The areola and nipple are distinctly projecting from the mound of breast tissue. The areola has a noticeable darker coloration, and so do the nipples. This stage usually takes place between the ages of 12 and 13.

- *Stage five:* This is the mature adult breast with a distinct breast mound, fully formed nipple and areola. This usually happens around a girl's 13th birthday. Breasts continue to grow throughout the teenage years and the final growth usually takes place by the age of 18 or 19.

OK. Now that we've told you all this wonderful scientific stuff about the very distinct series of stages of breast development, you shouldn't be surprised when we tell you that girls go back and forth between stages and that it isn't a straight line from flat chest to beautiful womanly breasts. For instance, a girl involved in serious athletic competitions can have some stage reversal or even stop having periods for awhile.

Hormonal fluctuations can make a girl's budding breasts look like Stage 3 one day and Stage 2 the next and perhaps Stage 4 a week later, then back to Stage 3. Don't stress over it. This is perfectly normal.

Since we're guessing pretty much that 10- and 11-year old girls aren't reading this book and their Moms and Grandmas are, you'll probably remember that there were days of extreme breast tenderness and then it would pass. Many girls complain about tenderness and even pain. This is because the mammary glands are developing and sometimes they grow very fast. This can actually last for two years or more. Many women complain of breast tenderness before their menstrual periods throughout their reproductive lives.

Also, as a girl approaches the time when her menstrual periods begin, usually somewhere between Tanner Stages 3 and 4, (but not always), estrogen and other female hormones become a major factor in literally every aspect of her life.

A few words about puberty

KATHLEEN SAYS: This is my personal passion and I hope sharing some of this information with you will help you and your family live long healthy lives.

Thelarche and menarche, the scientific terms for the changes that take place over several years of a young girl's life, combine in a mix of changes to her body that we loosely term puberty.

Yet there is cause to be concerned. The average American girl now reaches menarche a full 18 months earlier than girls of just 50 years ago.

A landmark 1997 study of 17,000 girls startled parents with its findings that nearly 7 percent of white girls and 27 percent of black girls started developing breasts by age 7 - during second grade.

In fact, pediatricians are no longer alarmed about breast tissue growth among girls under the age of 2. I was amazed when I discovered my 21-month old granddaughter was developing a breast on one side! Her pediatrician told my daughter this is "fairly common" among little girls. But in girls who were not yet even two years old? I was horrified.

Many experts theorize that this condition, which now has a medical name — "precocious puberty" — is caused by xenoestrogens. These are toxins that act like estrogen in the human body and unbalance the delicate dance of hormones.

Many of these hormone disruptors are petrochemical-based and have been found in a multitude of common household plastics, including the toddler's best friend, Sippy cups. They're also found in pesticides, dioxin, food dyes, preservatives and even in common cosmetics. Among the most dangerous xenoestrogens are phthalates (pronounced THAL-aytz) that are used to soften plastics.

We are all exposed to them all the time. They have also worked their way into the water supply by becoming airborne (as industrial air pollutants) or in agricultural chemicals leeching through the ground into the water supply.

Growth hormones injected into dairy cattle have brought hormone disruptors into our milkstream and, to a certain degree, into our meat supply.

These xenoestrogens became part of our environment about 70 years ago. Their effects have been profound. Xenoestrogens disrupt the process of reproduction, causing low sperm count in boys and early puberty in girls. Phthalates are also known to increase the risk of breast cancer.

Prevention is the best path. Here are a few suggestions:

- *Go organic with dairy:* Organic dairy products are a must for all children who have been weaned from breast milk. The hormonal risks and those posed by the antibiotics used in non-organic dairy operations are very large.

- *Go organic entirely, if you can:* This is not just for kids, it's for all ages. The harsh chemicals used in food production, processing and preservation are immensely harmful to everyone's health. If your budget will tolerate it, buy as many organic products as possible, from your meats to your fruits, vegetables, grains, cleaning products, even cosmetics and personal care items like soap and shampoo.

- *Eliminate pesticides and herbicides from your lawn:* The vast majority of these toxic chemicals consumed in America today are used by homeowners and they are often used incorrectly. If you must use them, follow all the precautions, wear gloves, masks and measure precisely the amounts you need. Store them safely and away from your house, garden and water supply.

- *Banish plastic from your house:* We know this is nearly impossible. But as much as possible, don't buy food packaged in plastic because the phthalates leech into the food, especially in meat that is packaged on Styrofoam trays and wrapped in plastic wrap. Don't drink out of plastic cups and don't let your kids do so either unless they are made from polyethylene designated #2HDPE or #4HDPE. Paper cups are still very much available. Never heat food in a microwave in plastic containers because that accelerates the phthalate leeching. While you're at it, get rid of any Teflon-coated cookware. At high heat it puts off gasses and harmful chemicals known to cause various types of cancer. Opt instead for cast iron, or better yet, porcelain-coated cast iron.

- *Banish plastic and Styrofoam from your life as much as you can.* We're specifically talking about drinking hot liquids out of Styrofoam cups like that lovely latte at your favorite java house. The fumes from the hot liquid interacting with petrochemical-based Styrofoam are very toxic—and you're putting the cup to your mouth, so you inhale them with every sip! Avoid bottled water for the same reasons: not only is the waste a huge burden on the environment, the plastic bottle leeches phthalates into the water. The leeching is accelerated if the bottle is left in a warm place, like your car or your gym bag. Opt for a good water filter at home and carry your water with you in glass or high quality polyethylene containers that won't leech.

Protecting yourself from xenoestrogens as much as possible is important for every human being, but it is especially crucial for children and women of all ages.

EFFECTS OF UNBALANCED ESTROGEN

- Increases risk of breast cancer
- Increases risk of endometrial cancer
- Stimulates breast cysts
- Increases body fat storage
- Causes salt and fluid retention
- Causes depression
- Causes headaches
- Interferes with thyroid hormones
- Greatly increases the risk of stroke
- Decreases libido (sex drive)
- Hampers control of healthy blood sugar levels
- Causes loss of zinc
- Causes the retention of unhealthy levels of copper
- Reduces oxygen levels in all cells

Reaching womanhood

There was once a time when girls were celebrated with a special ceremony when they came into womanhood. There were gifts, celebrations and words of wisdom passed from older women to the new woman. There were new responsibilities and new privileges as well. In those ancient times, marriage and motherhood often followed quickly and with them all the burdens that raising a family placed on a young woman. But of course, those were times when life expectancy was much shorter. We should be glad that in modern times, there is not such a rush to preserve the human race.

Yet the celebration of the transition from maidenhood to womanhood was, in those times, recognition of the beauty, grace and potential of a woman's body. Young women were taught to be proud of their bodies and to honor their new curves and crevices.

In today's world, sexuality sometimes comes too early and is tied up in many societal pressures that keep young women from fully blossoming into their healthy sexual identities. While their bodies may be ready and eager for all the joys of womanhood, today's young women would be well counseled to take the time to let their emotional maturity catch up with their newfound physical maturity. Dr. Ben likes to counsel young women to nurture a strong sense of self-esteem so they wait until they fall in love and let their first sexual experience be within the bonds of marriage, rather than letting society pressure them into it before they are ready.

We think it is society's misfortune that this custom of celebrating a girl's passage into womanhood has been lost. Perhaps if we once again adopt the tradition of honoring our girls as they become women, problems of eating disorders, low self-esteem and the age-old question "Am I good enough?" will begin to fade from the collective female consciousness.

A woman's breast

This seems like a no brainer, since it is the ordinary woman that goes through a stage lasting 20 to 30 years when her breasts remain more or less the same except during pregnancy.

We can't emphasize enough how important it is to know your breasts well. This is the only way you can tell if there are changes that merit medical attention.

During each menstrual cycle, breast tissue tends to swell because of changes in the body's levels of estrogen and progesterone. The milk glands and ducts enlarge, and in turn, the breasts retain water. During menstruation, breasts may temporarily feel swollen, painful, tender, or lumpy. That's why the monthly breast self-examination (BSE) is best done shortly after the end of your period when your breasts are less tender and don't feel so bumpy.

Breast changes during pregnancy

When you are pregnant, your breasts undergo several changes. That's why it's important for your doctor to do a thorough breast exam during your first prenatal office visit, so you can establish a baseline or an idea of what your breasts are like as they undergo the routine changes of pregnancy. Your breasts should be examined on every monthly prenatal visit.

During pregnancy, a variety of breast changes occur. Typically, breasts become tender and the nipples become sore a few weeks after conception. The breasts also increase in size very quickly. It is not uncommon for a woman's breasts to increase by one or two cup sizes during and after pregnancy. The most rapid period of breast growth is during the first eight weeks of pregnancy.

The Montgomery's glands surrounding the areola (pigmented region around the nipple) becomes darker and more prominent, and the areola itself darkens. The nipples also become larger and more erect as they prepare for milk production and the sucking baby. The blood vessels within the breast enlarge as surges of estrogen stimulate the growth of the ducts and surges of progesterone cause the glandular tissue to expand.

Two hormones are responsible for milk production: prolactin and oxytocin. Prolactin is sometimes referred to as the "mothering hormone" because some people believe it also causes a calming effect that makes women feel more maternal. The body begins producing prolactin approximately eight weeks after conception. As the pregnancy progresses, the levels of prolactin steadily increase, peaking at the time of birth. As her body produces more and more prolactin, high levels of estrogen and progesterone block some of the prolactin receptors and stop milk production from taking place until after the baby is born.

After birth, estrogen and progesterone levels decrease and the production of prolactin declines. Breasts will usually begin to produce milk three to five days after the birth. During these few days before milk is produced, the body produces colostrum, a liquid substance that contains antibodies and growth hormones to help protect the baby against infections. Some physicians believe that colostrum also decreases an infant's chances of developing asthma and other allergies. Within a few days, the infant's own immune system becomes more self-sufficient and colostrum will no longer be produced.

The other hormone responsible for milk production, oxytocin, delivers the milk that prolactin has produced. When an infant suckles at the mother's breast, it brings milk out of the nipples. This suction signals the body to make more milk (using prolactin) and deliver more milk (using oxytocin). The body also produces a variety of other hormones (insulin, thyroid, and cortisol) that provide the infant with nutrition from the mother's milk. A woman's body will continue to produce milk until she stops breast feeding, and even then, it may take several months for milk production to completely stop. The breasts will usually return to their previous size (or slightly smaller) when she stops breast-feeding.

Breast changes after menopause

When a woman reaches menopause (typically in her late 40s or early 50s), her body's production of estrogen and progesterone, decreases dramatically. Even in the years before menopause, the time called perimenopause, the levels of these hormones may fluctuate wildly. The fluctuating hormones cause a variety of symptoms in many women including hot flashes, night sweats, mood changes, difficulty concentrating, vaginal dryness and insomnia.

During this time, the breasts also undergo changes. For some women, the breasts become more tender and lumpy, sometimes forming cysts (accumulated pockets of fluid).

The glandular tissue in the breasts, which has been kept firm so that the glands could produce milk, shrinks after menopause and is replaced with fatty tissue. The breasts also tend to increase in size and sag because the fibrous connective tissue loses its strength.

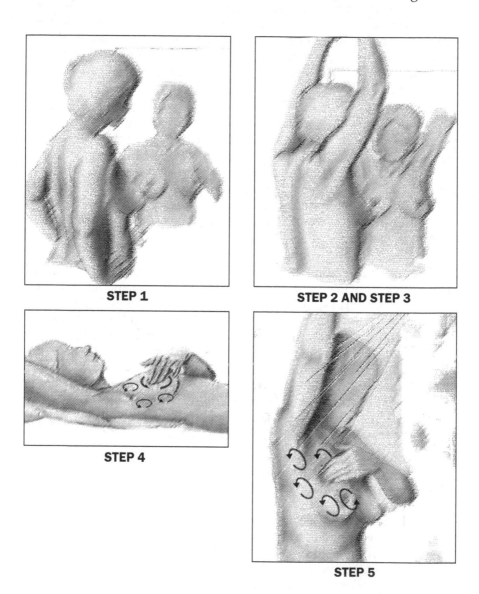

STEP 1

STEP 2 AND STEP 3

STEP 4

STEP 5

Breast self-exams

Remember back at the beginning of this chapter we said it is important for you to know your breasts well so you can detect changes?

Undoubtedly you've heard of breast self-examinations (BSEs) and hopefully you are religiously performing them every month. Wouldn't it be wonderful if every mom taught her daughter how to do a BSE as one of the ways she can be welcomed into womanhood?

For women who are in their menstrual years, it's a good idea to do your BSE the week after your period ends. Your breasts will be less tender at that time and some of the fullness and lumpiness that can be caused by estrogen will be less pronounced.

If you are no longer menstruating, choose a day and do your BSE the same day every month. It's easy to remember if you do it the first of the month.

Remember our discussion of what's "normal?" What's normal is what's normal for you. Whatever you have is normal for you. You need to know what's normal for you and be very familiar with your breasts. You might want to do a little breast map on a piece of notebook paper. Show the curves, shape, and nipples. You might even want to use a ruler to measure any cysts or lumps. Then when you refer to it every month, you won't have to rely on memory.

Before we get to the refresher course, we want to address something that Dr. Ben has heard hundreds of times in response to his question about whether a patient is regularly doing her BSEs. "I don't do them because I'm afraid of what I might find," they tell him.

Now, we know our readers are intelligent women and we know that you know this doesn't make sense. Don't let fear sabotage you.

If you can't bring yourself to do your BSE, delegate! Ask your husband or boyfriend. We're sure you'll have an enthusiastic helper!

If you are doing those all-important BSEs, congratulations! Here's a refresher course. If you're not, there's no better time than now to start. It's simple and it only takes a few minutes a month.

The five steps of a breast self-examination

Step 1: Begin by standing in front of a mirror, your hands on your hips. Look for:

- Breasts that are their usual size, shape, and color.
- Breasts that are evenly shaped without visible distortion or swelling.

If you see any of the following changes, bring them to your doctor's attention:

- Dimpling, puckering, or bulging of the skin.
- A nipple that has changed position or a nipple that has become inverted (pushed inward instead of sticking out) since your last BSE.
- Redness, soreness, rash, or swelling.

Step 2: Now, raise your arms over your head and look for the same changes.

Step 3: Move your arms up over your head and then bring your hands behind your back. The movement of your nipples should be synchronized – that means they should go in the same direction at the same time with the natural movement of your body.

Step 4: Next, lie down on your back with one arm behind your head. Use your right hand to feel your left breast and then your left hand to feel your right breast. Use a firm, smooth touch with the first few fingers of your hand, keeping the fingers flat and together. It's important to keep your fingers on the skin and move them across the breast without lifting them to be sure you don't miss any spots.

It helps to use some massage oil or a light almond oil to help take the air space out from between the skin and the fingers and make the exam easier. It also makes your fingers more sensitive and helps them to pick up information better.

Always start at the same place. Be very systematic, do the same routine each time. Be sure to check in your armpits since that's where 90 percent of the drainage of the breast goes and there are lots of lymph nodes. Remember, what you have felt every month is normal for you.

Make little bitty circles about a half inch in diameter with your fingertips while you make a great big circle around the entire breast.

The armpits are a great place to start your exam. Just continue downward in an arch to where the bra hits your chest below the breast and then up and around to the sternum (breast bone), up the sternum to the collar bone then continuing over to the armpit where we began. You'll be making little circles all the time with your fingers. Now we have made this complete circle around the outside of the breast, continue in smaller and smaller circles covering the entire breast until you get to the nipple.

Now we are going to check for nipple discharge. Place your fingers about three inches away from the nipple. Press down and move the fingers toward the nipple. Repeat this for all four quadrants of the breast. Gently squeeze each nipple between your finger and thumb and check for nipple discharge.

A very slight amount of nipple discharge is not unusual. It could be a milky or yellow fluid or blood. There may even be a black discharge. It looks a little scary, but it's a fungus that lives happily and harmlessly in the breasts of many women. A bloody discharge is significant and should not be ignored. A black discharge is worth following up with your doctor, but it is nothing to panic about.

If you are small breasted (a B cup or smaller), you'll be circling the entire breast first on the skin surface and then again with more pressure, about half an inch deep into the breast tissue. If you have larger breasts (a C cup or larger), do one more complete circuit on a third level about an inch into the breast tissue.

Step 5: Finally, feel your breasts while you are standing or sitting. Many women find that the easiest way to feel their breasts is when their skin is wet, so they like to do this step in the shower. Cover your entire breast, using the same hand movements described in Step 4.

OK. So you found something new

First and foremost: DO NOT PANIC. Breasts are changeable and there are many times when your breasts may feel lumpy or bumpy.

If you have found something that concerns you, fear is not the appropriate response. The appropriate response is to investigate and find out what is going on.

If you find a spot that is tender or squishy, it's most likely a cyst. These are rarely malignant, but they are cause for a consultation with your doctor.

A small hard painless mass the size of a pea or larger may be cause for concern. See your doctor.

Panicking won't help. Deciding to "wait and see" is not the answer either. Sound medical advice at an early stage can make a large difference.

Dr. Ben listens carefully when a woman tells him she has found something suspicious. Women have an innate knowledge of their bodies and know when there is something wrong.

You'll probably be asked to have a mammogram or a thermogram, an ultrasound or a biopsy. We'll be discussing the upsides and the downsides of these and other diagnostic tools in the next chapter. Your doctor may also want to do a biopsy by taking a small tissue sample from the lump. Do some more reading before you proceed with a biopsy. We'll be discussing this in detail in Chapter 8.

Remember the odds are in your favor. Most breast lumps - as many as four out of five biopsied – are benign (noncancerous). Nevertheless, you can only be sure if you see your doctor and check it out.

Many women have breasts that feel very lumpy and bumpy. Others have breasts that are smooth and evenly textured throughout. Just a little bumpiness is not reason for panic—it is the changes that warrant your attention and you can only know if there are changes if you're doing your regular exams.

If you tend to have lumpy or tender breasts, you might consider avoiding caffeine, nicotine, theophylline (found in tea) and chocolate, since all are thought to influence breast lumpiness.

Chapter 3 # THE ESSENTIALS OF BREAST HEALTH

Commit yourself to the health of your breasts today. That commitment on the part of many women, dare we say most women, is based on fear. Fear that something is wrong. If you try not to think about your breasts, touch them or care for them in other ways because you are afraid that you'll find something wrong, think about the Law of Attraction and think about changing your thinking. Then do it.

In the last chapter, you learned about the basics of breast anatomy and how to do the all-important breast self-exam (BSE).

Now it's time to learn how to take the protective measures that will keep your breasts healthy. They, for the most part, parallel the guidelines for general good health.

Free movement

We're not throwbacks to the 60s, and we don't recommend bra burning, because bras can be valuable pieces of apparel at least for social and athletic purposes. However, we ask you to consider keeping your bra for public consumption and going braless in the comfort of your own home.

There are three major reasons why bras can be contrary to breast health:

- They raise the temperature of the breasts.
- They restrict oxygen and nutrient flow to the tissues.
- They restrict the flow of toxin-removing lymphatic fluids.

While the medical community has not yet made a definite pronouncement, Dr. Ben is convinced that there is sufficient research to prove there is a connection between wearing a bra and a woman's risk of breast cancer.

Let's start with a few sobering numbers.

Sydney Ross Singer and Soma Grismaijer, husband and wife authors of Dressed to Kill (Avery Press, 1995), interviewed 4,730 women in five major US cities between 1991 and 1993. Their findings were very impressive:

- Women who wore their bras for 24 hours per day had a 3 out of 4 chance of developing breast cancer in their lifetimes. (The study included 2056 subjects for the cancer group and 2674 for the standard group).

- Women who wore bras more than 12 hours per day, but not to bed, had a 1 in 7 risk of developing breast cancer.

- Women who wore their bras less than 12 hours per day had a 1 out of 152 risk.

- Women who wore bras rarely or never, had a 1 in 168 chance of getting breast cancer.

While there has been little follow-up research, we are confident that someday we'll know why this study showed a 125-fold difference in cancer rates between bra-free breasts and those constricted and heated by 24-hour-per-day bra-wearing.

There are lots of puzzle pieces to put in place here and we're aware that there may be some leaps of logic. Direct clinical research simply does not exist and probably never will exist. That's because drug companies fund research on new drugs that can make them money and they cannot make money on lifestyle changes that may prevent cancer.

There are many causes of breast cancer, but since we believe wearing a bra is one of them, it's one risk that can very easily be addressed.

Breast temperature

Let's go back to our anatomy lesson for just a few paragraphs.

Certain parts of the human body, including breasts, testicles and penises, were designed to be appendages, or parts that protrude outside the body. They are designed to flourish in a cooler environment than the usual 98.6 degree body temperature, give or take a degree or two.

We know that cancer cells thrive in warmer temperatures and we know that warmer temperatures can alter hormone function. Since breast cancer is a hormone dependent type of uncontrolled cell growth, it stands to reason that if we have a piece of clothing that insulates the breasts and generally keeps them warmer than they would be if they were uncovered, we might have a problem.

There haven't been many studies on these issues, so science hasn't yet caught up with common sense, but intuitively, it makes sense to us.

We do know that males who have an undescended testicle (it stays hotter than it was designed to because it is lodged inside the abdominal cavity) have a much higher risk of cancer in that testicle.

It's been nearly 30 years since Dr. John Douglas of the Southern California Permanente Medical Center suggested that women who wear bras have a higher risk of breast cancer. In his medical practice and the examination of several hundred women, Douglas observed that the heavier the bra material, the warmer a woman's breasts would be and women who did not wear bras or wore them occasionally had generally cooler breasts.

While there hasn't been much interest in the subject since then, two British breast surgeons more recently studied 100 women with breast pain to determine if they would improve if they went braless. Half the women found their pain was significantly reduced after going braless for three months.

Researchers theorized that going bra-free not only lowers the temperature of the breasts, but decreases the risk of breast cancer.

Decreased oxygen flow

Those red marks left behind by your bra are signs that circulation is being impaired. If blood flow is decreased, the supply of nutrients and oxygen to the tissues of the breast is decreased. This is not a healthy thing.

We'll be talking a great deal more about Otto Warburg, a German doctor and researcher who won the Nobel Prize in medicine in 1931 for his work that showed decreased oxygen flow actually causes cancer cells to grow. It's amazing to us that this German genius actually found the cause of most types of cancer more than 85 years ago!

Let's back up just a little bit for a moment.

You may or may not know that each cell actually has to breathe, to bring in oxygen and nutrient molecules so it can perform its designated function.

Dr. Warburg discovered that cancer cells invariably thrive in an anaerobic environment, one where the oxygen has been cut off. This can happen in a number of ways, including when the blood and lymphatic flow is restricted for any reason.

You may have heard that an acid pH is the cause of cancer. Acid pH and decreased oxygen flow are one and the same. Scientifically, this is called the oxygen-hemoglobin disassociation curve. Translation: As the blood becomes more acidic, the oxygen cannot disconnect from its carrier, the hemoglobin molecules in the blood. The oxygen saturation of the blood might be 100 percent, but the cells can be starving for oxygen if the pH is too acid.

Lymphatic constriction

The lymphatic system is a major component of the immune system. Its nodes, vessels, ducts, tissues and capillaries return excess fluid to the circulatory system. It transports fluids, fatty acids and forms immune cells.

The lymph nodes surround the breast tissue and spread around into the armpits. The entire lymphatic system is, for all practical purposes, an alternate type of circulatory system that is designed to sweep toxins out of your body and strengthen your immune system. It collaborates with white blood cells in lymph nodes to protect the body from being infected by cancer cells, fungi, viruses or bacteria.

Women's breasts are meant to move with every step. Every little bounce of the breast while walking, running, twisting or turning actually gently massages the breast and stimulates the lymphatic flow.

Wearing a bra, particularly one with constricting underwires, prevents that normal lymphatic flow and allows toxins to accumulate in and around the breast tissues, exactly where you don't want them to be. Our friends who practice Chinese medicine are also concerned about the metal and pressure on the biomeridians from underwire bras.

We know that pregnancy and breast feeding help develop the lymphatic system surrounding the breasts. Specifically, pregnancies before age 21 and breast feeding for at least one year can decrease future cancer risks.

We also know that women of higher income groups have higher incidences of breast cancer. Perhaps one of the factors in that statistic might be that professional women have a greater tendency to wear bras for a longer period of time each day.

We also know that women who exercise have a lower risk factor. Better lymphatic circulation and more breast movement may be providing protection.

BREAST MASSAGE

Breast massage is important for stimulating lymphatic flow, circulation and good breast health.

The technique is simple:

- Take off your bra, if you're wearing one.
- Rub your breasts in a circular motion
- Rotate them in opposite directions.
- Continue for 3 to 5 minutes.

That's it! Do this at least once daily and your breasts and your body will thank you. Several brief massages during the day would also be very beneficial. It's easily accomplished, in the privacy of your car, or in the bathroom. Just take 30 seconds. Yes, it is OK to touch your breasts. This is about your health.

Large breasts and back pain

Surprisingly, going braless actually reduces back pain in large breasted women. We know that seems a bit counter-intuitive, but it's the bra, not the breasts, that causes the back pain according to a study published in the Clinical Journal of Pain. It seems that women with back pain who were advised to go braless or wear a strapless bra for two weeks achieved almost complete relief from the debilitating pain. In fact, 79 percent were so happy with the results that they decided to ditch their bras permanently.

Think of the women who contemplate extensive, painful and potentially dangerous breast reduction surgery because of the back pain associated with large breasts. It's worth a safe and simple experiment in bra-lessness.

Worried about sagging?

No woman wants to sag. There is simply too much societal pressure to have high, perky breasts.

But going braless may actually stimulate the muscles around your breasts to become stronger and more self-supporting. A 1991 Japanese study suggests that not only were braless women better able to hold their own, but that the anti-sagging effect was more pronounced in large-breasted women.

Social convention

Social convention is certainly a valid factor in your decision whether to wear a bra or not. Societal pressure goes counter to bouncing breasts, especially in a business setting. If you are concerned about your nipples showing, you might want to try a camisole. There are even some very comfortable ones with very light bra inserts that may satisfy social convention as well as keeping your breasts healthy.

Large-breasted women certainly are under more pressure from this angle than their smaller-breasted sisters.

It's your choice, and it's not only your physical health, but your emotional comfort that is at stake.

If you choose to continue to wear a bra during the day, we urge you to take it off when you get home and certainly, never to wear a bra to bed.

We also urge you to be properly fitted for any bra you decide to wear. A good fit will minimize circulatory and lymphatic constriction.

Is it possible to find a bra that fits?

Yes, believe it or not, it is possible to find a bra that fits well and is comfortable. Most women suffer from wearing poorly fitted bras.

If you've decided to continue to wear a bra at least part of the time, it is essential to have one that fits well and does not bind or constrict you. It's also important to look for a bra that is made of the most lightweight fabric possible for ventilation or cotton for absorbency in sports bras. Both will minimize the insulating factor.

The ideal way to get a bra that fits properly is to go to a large department store that has a lingerie department and ask for a lingerie specialist to help fit you. There actually are such places and people who are trained to do the job very precisely. An added advantage is that you can try on several styles until you find one that suits you best.

Here is an easy formula if you want to do the measuring on your own. These measurements should be taken without clothing unless there is significant sagging, then you'll need to wear your best fitting bra to get a measurement. You'll need a helper since the measurements should be taken while you are standing normally with your arms at your sides:

1. *Chest measurement:* Place a cloth measuring tape under your breasts. Wrap the tape around your body so the tape measure meets the beginning part of the tape. When you have the measurement number, add five inches –or three inches if your measurement is more than 33 inches — to get the band size. If your result is an odd number, round it

up to the next even number. The band should fit snugly, but you should be able to slide your hand beneath the back comfortably.

2. *Bust measurement:* Next, you will measure around your chest at the largest or fullest part of your breasts, called your "bustline." You need to measure with your arms straight down, so ask someone you feel comfortable with to help you.

3. *Cup size:* Your bust measurement will be higher than your chest measurement. Your cup size is the difference between your chest measurement and your bustline measurement.

Here's a chart to help you determine cup size:

DIFFERENCE	CUP SIZE
½ inch	AA
1 inch	A
2 inches	B
3 inches	C
4 inches	D
5 inches	DD or E
6 inches	F or EE
7 inches	G or EEE

As you well know by now, every woman's breasts are different, so use this chart as a guideline, not a gospel. Get an idea of the size you need and then try on several bras to determine what works best for you.

DR. BEN SAYS: I rarely frequent the lingerie department, but I have seen enough bras in my medical career to know that most of them are about as flexible and about as comfortable as a suit of armor, and many fit just about as well.

If I could design the perfect bra, it would be a shelf-like garment made of lightweight and absorbent material that supports the breast from underneath, without wires. It would not cover the nipple or the top of the breast so the breast tissue wouldn't get too warm. It would support the Cooper's ligaments that follow the contours of the breast from the top and the bottom so they will not get stretched out. The straps would be wide and well-padded to keep weight off the shoulders. I think this actually would be healthy and a great joy to women who have suffered from wearing uncomfortable bras for most of their adult lives.

KATHLEEN SAYS: Just looking at the above material was enough to convince me. As I was sitting at my desk writing this section, I stripped off my bra the moment I saw the research about wearing bras and breast cancer risk. Yes, I'll still wear a bra for social reasons, but since I work at home, that means I'll put one on only a couple of times a week. I'll also wear it when I ride my horse since cantering can be downright painful without some support.

Leaving my bra in the drawer doesn't bother me a bit, since I have always suspected that the person who invented the bra was a masochist or sadist or both, depending on whether or not you believe the legend that this particular garment was invented by a woman.

Breathe

This may seem almost laughably obvious, but oxygenating your system through deep and regular breathing is an excellent way of keeping all your cells healthy and avoiding the oxygen-starved environment that fosters the growth of cancer cells.

When you are breathing rapidly, you are also exhaling more carbon dioxide, which raises the pH and gives you a healthier alkaline environment.

Deep, slow yogic or abdominal type breaths are healthy for your body, as are the deep breathing that accompanies exercise.

Better off without antiperspirants

There has long been concern that aluminum in products like cookware and antiperspirant deodorants might contribute to Alzheimer's disease, but newer research connects antiperspirants with breast cancer as well.

The primary lymph nodes in the armpits carry toxins out of your body by several methods, including perspiration. One theory about the association between breast cancer and antiperspirant use is that the lymph nodes are not allowed to do their job properly. Another theory is that the aluminum in the antiperspirants interferes with estrogen action and possibly even changes the cellular matrix of breast cells. It is certainly telling that the majority of breast cancers occur in the upper outer quadrants of the breast. Since that's the place closest to the armpit, it's enough for us to recommend that you change your deodorant if you're using antiperspirants.

Take a good look at the label and reject anything with aluminum chlorhydrate. There are many natural deodorants on the market that work very well without aluminum. Kathleen particularly likes the deodorant crystals that are long lasting, antibacterial and best of all, aluminum free.

Exercise

There are many compelling reasons to have a regular exercise program.

Aerobic exercise will certainly improve your breathing and bring loads of oxygen into your body.

It also brings about that all-important bounce that helps with lymphatic flow, as we mentioned earlier in this chapter.

What's more, exercise will literally extend your life. Scientific research shows that those who exercise regularly, even if they don't start until middle-age, can actually reduce their risk of dying from any cause by nearly 25 percent.

Plus, a 14-year Norwegian study involving 25,000 women found that those who exercised at least four hours a week had a 37 percent lower risk of developing breast cancer than inactive women.

But you hate exercise, you say? Unless you're a complete couch potato, there must be some form of exercise you enjoy. You may not even think of it as exercise. How about dancing? Gardening? Playing tag with your kids or tossing the Frisbee to the dog?

In fact, gardening is one of the most effective forms of exercise known. It burns even more calories (480 an hour) than jogging and works all your muscle groups. Kathleen finds gardening particularly enjoyable and a relaxing form of exercise.

Even some of the less enjoyable household activities like vacuuming, dusting, bending, straightening clutter, hauling kids up the stairs, folding laundry or grocery shopping count as exercise.

Your goal should be to get five hours of exercise a week, spread over at least five days. It doesn't count if you go out on Saturday afternoon for a 30-mile run and do nothing the rest of the week. You'll probably injure yourself.

We can hear groans. We feel your pain.

Here's the key to a successful exercise program: You've got to love it.

We don't mean you've got to like it or tolerate it or you'll grudgingly do it because it's good for you. Find something you really love and you'll do it for a lifetime. Unless you are committed to exercise for a lifetime, your program and all your good intentions will fall away like a New Year's resolution in February.

Do some searching. If you're the type who likes lots of people around you, by all means, sign up for a gym membership. If you love peace and quiet, solitary early morning walks may become your passion.

Maybe you're more the type to enjoy joining a hiking group or a volleyball league, a ballroom dancing class or a yoga class. These are all great forms of exercise.

More solitary forms of exercise might include cycling, swimming and practicing that yoga you learned in class.

Walking is perfectly sufficient, if you love it.

Recent research suggests that intensity of exercise is not as important as we once thought. That means an after dinner stroll with your sweetheart or taking the stairs instead of the elevator or even quietly walking in place while you are on the telephone can add up those minutes in small increments that won't leave you gasping for breath and pouring sweat. And all of them count toward your hour-a day. Maybe you'll want to kick it up on the weekend with a longer hike or with sprint races against your kids in the local pool.

When we begin to think of exercise in broader terms, it's easier to get in that five hours a week.

We mentioned the use of bras earlier in this chapter and the message bears repeating here: Less is better. For some women, especially those who are large-breasted, running, cantering on a horse or playing basketball may be downright painful without a good support bra. Wear a good cotton support bra for your exercise sessions, and then take it off as soon as possible afterward.

Try several forms of exercise and see what fits best for you.

Also feel free to change things up. Don't do the same exercise all the time or you will get bored. If you get bored, you'll drop it, and that's what we want to avoid at all costs.

If you can get yourself really excited about two forms of exercise, so much the better, because they will work different parts of your body.

Among its myriad benefits, exercise is an excellent mood elevator and stress reliever.

THE BEST EXERCISE YOU CAN DO IN AN HOUR	
ACTIVITY	CALORIES BURNED
Aerobics	422
Exercise bike	392
Dancing	317
Tai Chi	281
Walking dog	246

Manage stress

The Centers for Disease Control and Prevention says 85 percent of all illness is caused by stress. Some experts say that figure should be as high as 95 percent.

Unless you live in a cave in the Himalayas, it is impossible to exist in today's world without stress. We all feel it: The pressures of a job, home, kids, health and finances. It goes on and on. And now we're lucky enough to have cell phones, so _____ (fill in the blank here: your office, your kids, your spouse, your best friend in crisis, your child's teacher) can reach you any time, any place.

Every day, our personal time shrinks. We consider it an indulgence if we can squeeze in the time to simply sit and enjoy a cup of tea or read a book for the sheer pleasure of it, or take a long leisurely bubble bath.

Never before in history have humans had so much to do and so many varieties of ways to do it. Even sitting around the television set at night with your family can be stress-producing with so many channels from which to choose, so much violence and fast paced action.

Call these the vagaries of modern lifestyle. Whether it's the chicken or the egg, we can't really tell you, but we live in a fast-paced, noisy world. From high-speed Internet to fast food to the fast-track in schools and careers, we rarely get a chance to catch our collective breath. It's taking a huge toll on our health.

A recent survey shows 75 percent all women feel "great stress" at least one day a week.

Unfortunately, unresolved stress in your life can lead to a downward spiral of disease conditions that can be dramatically harmful to your health.

We're getting closer to the chapter on *The Healing Codes*™, but we'll plant this seed in your mind: Since stress is at the core of most disease, resolving your stress is the key to healing.

Unresolved stress, the kind of stress you haven't dealt with and eliminated from your body and mind, is sometimes called toxic stress. This sustained stress overrides your body's natural abilities to bounce back, keeping stress hormone levels high and suppressing your immune system.

The Healing Codes™ are the best possible way of managing your stress, but you can also insert tools into your daily life that will help.

Finding time for yourself for rest and quiet may seem impossible, but you can do it if you get creative about it.

Kathleen has a friend whose husband takes charge of their two rambunctious toddlers every day for an hour after he gets home from work so she can have a bubble bath or read a book or take a nap. It's done a world of good for their relationship as a couple and as a family, not to speak of Mom's mental and physical health.

A big stress reducer is that powerful two-letter word: NO. It doesn't have to be mean spirited or angry, just firm. When the world in encroaching on too much of your time for your own well-being, it's time to consider saying, "No."

Birth Control

It's not nice to fool with Mother Nature. We were designed with intricate hormonal systems and feedback mechanisms for those hormones.

To put it simply, anytime you mess with those hormonal balances, you are going to cause problems.

Birth control pills, even if they are low estrogen doses, have wide-ranging effects on a woman including her ability to have an orgasm. The potency of the artificial estrogens is an issue because they override the natural balances in place in a woman's body. We know they effect glandular development related to breast tissue, and they increase the risk of blood clots, stroke and depression.

For that reason, we recommend you find alternate methods of birth control.

Condoms, IUDs and the rhythm method are safe, natural and effective methods of birth control that don't effect your hormones.

Supplements

We all need nutritional supplements. The depletion of the soil has made it impossible to get the nutrients we need from our food.

There are loads of supplements that are helpful in general, and we strongly urge you to take a good quality multi-vitamin every day. Be sure that it contains at least all of the RDA of the antioxidants vitamins A, C and E.

There are plenty of books on supplements, so we won't go into the other general health supplements, but we do want to give you some recommendations about supplements that are specifically beneficial for breast health.

Here are Dr. Ben's favorites:

D-Cholecalciferol: Articles about vitamin D are beginning to appear everywhere, suggesting that most of us are deficient in this essential vitamin and those deficiencies may be putting us at risk for cancer. This unique form of vitamin D is found in fish oil and it is the same type of vitamin D that humans formulate on their skin with the help of sunlight. One large study in the first National Health and Nutrition Examination Survey (NHANES I) found that adequate sunlight exposure and dietary vitamin D reduced the risk of breast cancer 20 years later. Another huge study of 88,000 women found that higher intakes of vitamin D were associated with significantly lower breast cancer risk in premenopausal women.

Calcium d-glucarate: New research links glucarate, a non-toxic substance produced in the body and certain fruits and vegetables, to cancer prevention. Glucarate plays a leading role in the process of glucuronidation, the body's way of ridding itself of potentially harmful carcinogens. Glucarate binds harmful toxins, carcinogens and excess estrogen together so the body can excrete them. Adding a supplement of calcium glucarate to your diet may be especially beneficial to help prevent breast cancer.

Indole-3 caribinol (I3C): This compound found in cruciferous vegetables (broccoli, cauliflower, brussel sprouts and cabbage) has well-substantiated research on its breast cancer pevention ability. I3C actually blocks harmful free estrogen molecules from hooking up with estrogen receptor sites on breast cells and decreases the risk of all types of estrogen-sensitive cancers, including breast, ovarian and uterine. It promotes the producation of estriol, the good estrogen.

L-methylfolate: Folic acid is known to suppress breast cancer and this form of folic acid is the most readily available for the body's use. Harvard research shows that women with the highest intake of folates had the lowest rates of breast cancer. It's particularly relevant for postmenopausal women. It is also known to help fetal brain and spinal cord development during pregnancy.

Phosphatidylcholine: This is another unique nutrient that has been shown to stop the spread of breast cancer by enhancing immune function. It is found in every living cell. It coats the nerves so they can function properly. It is essential for brain function and memory. It also protects the cardiovascular system.

Alpha Lipoic Acid: This compound may be the most powerful anti-oxidant ever discovered. Where vitamin C is only water soluble, and vitamin E is only fat soluble, ALA is both. It is the go-anywhere anti-oxidant that can quench the most potent free radicals. It also doubles as a renewing agent helping the body to recycle C, E, glutathione, and coenzyme Q10.

Red Wine Extract: The polyphenols in red wine are powerful antioxidants. Also called resveratrol, this exceptionally powerful cancer fighter has been found to stop cancer cells from beginning to grow, from clumping together into tumors and from spreading. It has been shown to be a potent force against breast cancer cells.

Probiotics: Adding these beneficial bacteria to your digestive system is a big step in shoring up your immune system's first line of defense. Unfortunately, most of the probiotic supplements currently being sold in the United States contain only two major strains of bacteria, Acidophilus and Bifidobacterium. We actually need about 500 different types of bacteria. Dr. Ben has quite successfully used a German product called Mutaflor®.

> DR. BEN SAYS: I want to say a few words about soy as a food and as a supplement. I know it's all the rage partly because of the plant estrogens it contains. Soy is generally considered a "safe" estrogen. Soy beans however cannot be consumed by humans without extensive processing and fermenting. Intuitively, I think there is something suspicious about this. The plant estrogens in soy do stimulate the human estrogen receptor sites, which act like electrical outlets that estrogen molecules can plug into. I think the jury is still out on whether they are healthy ones or not. I have never had a good feeling about soy and I wouldn't recommend using it as a supplement or consuming large amounts of it as a food.

Discuss these with your doctor

Finally, here are a few ideas to kick around with your doctor for breast health and gynecological common sense. They can make a huge difference in your breast health and your overall health:

- *Avoid antibiotics whenever possible.* Researchers found that women who took antibiotics for more than 500 days or who had more than 25 prescriptions in the course of a 17-year period more than doubled their risk of breast cancer compared with women who had not taken any antibiotics. This sounds like a huge amount of antibiotics and it is. Yet these kinds of dosages are fairly common in women treating acne, sinusitis or chronic infections. It's fine to use antibiotics if you really need them for a week or two to fight a serious bacterial infection. Don't take them for colds or flu, since they are useless against viruses and, if you use them too often, antibiotics may eventually stop working for you when you need them most.

- *Avoid chest X-rays unless they are absolutely necessary.* X-ray (including mammograms) expose you to radiation and radiation has time and time again been shown to cause cancer. This is especially risky in young women whose breasts are still developing. Unless there is a very serious reason to have a chest X-ray, refuse it, especially if you or your daughter are under the age of 18. If you know you are going to have an X-ray, load up on antioxidants. MRIs are great alternatives to X-rays and are almost always a preferable option.

- *Never let your doctor use a metal speculum.* They can transmit HPV (human papilloma virus), a sexually transmitted disease which causes cancer of the cervix and can be transmitted if the speculum is not sterilized perfectly. Insist on a disposable plastic speculum when you're having a pelvic exam.

Chapter 4 BALANCE THROUGH DIET AND LIFESTYLE

There are dozens of good books that will tell you to eat loads of fruits and vegetables for their abilities to neutralize free radical molecules that cause all kinds of diseases, including cancer. Yes, this is indeed true, but that is actually only part of the story.

Remember Dr. Otto Warburg, the 1931 winner of the Nobel Prize in medicine, the pioneer we mentioned a few pages back?

Well, not only did Dr. Warburg discover more than 85 years ago that all cancer cells have a unique ability to survive without oxygen, he also found that when body systems tip toward being more acidic in nature, the low oxygen environment they create promotes the growth of cancer cells.

It boggles the mind to think that more than 85 years ago we had the tools to conquer most types of cancer and that at the time, the medical profession recognized the validity of Dr., Warburg's research, but we've somehow forgotten all about it.

Normal cells that become cancerous have done so because of a low-oxygen, highly-acidic environment, among other factors.

Unless your body is in a slightly alkaline state, it cannot heal itself as well or protect itself from the cell mutations that become cancer.

If your body is becoming more acidic, among the first things you might notice are low energy and perhaps a tendency to get a lot of colds. When your body becomes more acidic, you might begin to experience headaches, aches, pains, stomach aches and joint pain. When the body becomes extremely acidic, the ability of the cells to take in oxygen diminishes. This is the ideal growing environment for cancer cells.

So how does your body become acidic and anaerobic?
The answers are pretty simple:

- By eating the Standard American Diet (SAD) which is heavy in sugar, processed foods, meat, dairy products and trans fats.
- By drinking acidic water.
- By smoking.
- By being stressed.

DR. BEN SAYS: I recommend a modified alkaline diet that is very different from the high protein, high fat, low carb diets that have recently become very popular. Most of all, I urge you to eat a sensible diet, heavy on alkalizing fruits and vegetables, healthy oils like fish oil and olive oil, and moderate amounts of animal products unless you have access to organically produced meats and dairy.

If your diet is heavy on animal products, sugar, alcohol, caffeine, trans fatty acids and processed foods, you have most likely tipped your system into the undesirable acidic state.

The modified alkaline diet

In order to maintain health, all of us want to be sensible and eat a diet that will nourish the whole body and especially keep breasts healthy. That is a sensible diet that contains a wealth of antioxidant-rich fruits and vegetables, complex carbohydrates like whole grains, legumes (dried beans), nuts, good fats and healthy meats.

If you remember your high school chemistry, pH measures the concentration of hydrogen in a solution. The more hydrogen, the more acidic it is (low pH); the less hydrogen, the more alkaline it is (high pH). The human body has a natural pH (acidity indicator) of 7.36 to 7.44, which is slightly alkaline.

If you have been eating the SAD (Standard American Diet), you are probably in an acidic state. How can you determine the state of acidity in your body? The simplest way is to get some pH paper (it's cheap — about $10 for 15 feet that will last you a year if you test daily) and test your urine and/or saliva.

The test is simple: Place the paper in your urine stream or in your mouth. The color will change. Simply compare the color to the master chart to let you know your pH reading.

It's best to take your reading early in the morning before you eat or drink anything. You can also take your reading in the afternoon at least two hours after you've had anything to eat or drink. Dr. Ben thinks saliva testing is slightly more accurate than urine testing, and, unless you have cancer, it's probably not necessary to test on a daily basis. Once or twice a week is sufficient.

Foods that keep your body in the optimal alkaline range are the ones that will keep your body in an optimum state of health.

How do you know if you have excess acidity in your diet and in your body? Here's a list of early symptoms:

- Low energy, chronic fatigue
- Excess mucous production
- Nasal congestion
- Frequent colds, flu, and infections
- Nervous, stressed, irritable, anxious, agitated
- Weak nails, dry hair, dry skin
- Formation of cysts, such as ovarian cysts, polycystic ovaries, benign breast cysts (fibrocystic breasts)
- Headaches
- Joint pain or arthritis
- Neuritis (nerve pain or numbness)
- Muscle pain
- Feeling better after a detox diet
- Hives and other allergic reactions
- Leg cramps and spasms
- Gastritis, acid indigestion

Probably most of us experience symptoms on this list from time to time. If you're experiencing them on a regular basis, it's time to alkalinize your diet, maximize your health and reduce your risk of cancer.

As a general guideline, the most valued foods on an alkaline diet are fruits and vegetables. Foods that you might consider acidic like lemons and tomatoes do not necessarily create an acidic effect on your body. In fact, these are excellent alkalizing foods.

This is a standard list of alkalinzing and acidifying foods. Individual needs vary, but a ratio of 75 percent alkalizing and 25 percent acidifying foods is recommended.

ALKALIZING FOODS

VEGETABLES
Garlic
Asparagus
Fermented Veggies
Watercress
Beets
Broccoli
Brussels sprouts
Cabbage
Carrot
Cauliflower
Celery
Chard
Chlorella
Collard Greens
Cucumber
Eggplant
Kale
Kohlrabi
Lettuce
Mushrooms
Mustard Greens
Dulce
Dandelions
Edible Flowers
Onions
Parsnips
   (high glycemic)
Peas
Peppers
Pumpkin
Rutabaga
Sea Veggies
Spirulina
Sprouts
Squashes
Alfalfa
Barley Grass
Wheat Grass
Wild Greens
Nightshade Veggies

SWEETENERS
Stevia

FRUITS
Apple
Apricot
Avocado
Banana
   (high glycemic)
Cantaloupe
Cherries
Currants
Dates/Figs
Grapes
Grapefruit
Lime
Honeydew Melon
Nectarine
Orange
Lemon
Peach
Pear
Pineapple
All Berries
Tangerine
Tomato
Tropical Fruits
Watermelon

PROTEIN
Eggs
Whey Protein Powder
Cottage Cheese
Chicken Breast
Yogurt
Almonds
Chestnuts
Tofu (fermented)
Flax Seeds
Pumpkin Seeds
Tempeh (fermented)
Squash Seeds
Sunflower Seeds
Millet
Sprouted Seeds
Nuts

OTHER
Apple Cider Vinegar
Bee Pollen
Lecithin Granules
Probiotic Cultures
Green Juices
Veggies Juices
Fresh Fruit Juice
Organic Milk
   (unpasteurized)
Mineral Water
Water
Green Tea
Herbal Tea
Dandelion Tea
Ginseng Tea
Banchi Tea
Kombucha

SPICES/ SEASONINGS
Cinnamon
Curry
Ginger
Mustard
Chili Pepper
Sea Salt
Miso
Tamari
All Herbs

ORIENTAL VEGETABLES
Maitake
Daikon
Dandelion Root
Shitake
Kombu
Reishi
Nori
Umeboshi
Wakame
Sea Veggies

ACIDIFYING FOODS

FATS & OILS
Avocado Oil
Canola Oil
Corn Oil
Hemp Seed Oil
Flax Oil
Lard
Olive Oil
Safflower Oil
Sesame Oil
Sunflower Oil

FRUITS
Cranberries

GRAINS
Rice Cakes
Wheat Cakes
Amaranth
Barley
Buckwheat
Corn
Oats (rolled)
Quinoi
Rice (all)
Rye
Spelt
Kamut
Wheat
Hemp Seed Flour

DAIRY
Cheese, Cow
Cheese, Goat
Cheese, Processed
Cheese, Sheep
Milk
Butter

NUTS & BUTTERS
Cashews
Brazil Nuts
Peanuts
Peanut Butter
Pecans
Tahini
Walnuts

ANIMAL PROTEIN
Beef
Carp
Clams
Fish
Lamb
Lobster
Mussels
Oyster
Pork
Rabbit
Salmon
Shrimp
Scallops
Tuna
Turkey
Venison

PASTA (WHITE)
Noodles
Macaroni
Spaghetti

OTHER
Distilled Vinegar
Wheat Germ
Potatoes
DRUGS & CHEMICALS
Chemicals
Drugs, Medicinal
Drugs, Psychedelic
Pesticides
Herbicides

ALCOHOL
Beer
Spirits
Hard Liquor
Wine

BEANS & LEGUMES
Black Beans
Chick Peas
Green Peas
Kidney Beans
Lentils
Lima Beans
Pinto Beans
Red Beans
Soy Beans
Soy Milk
White Beans
Rice Milk
Almond Milk

DR. BEN SAYS: I have a slightly different "take" on the alkaline diet because most charts do not take into consideration the benefits of organics. We've said it before, but the message bears repeating: Organic is best. I think that almost all organic foods move into the alkaline category, regardless of what these charts say. So, for example, if you consume organic nuts, chicken, beef, dairy products or whole grains in modest quantities, the foods will not upset your alkaline balance.

I think the acidity of meat products may be due to the antibiotics and hormones given to the animals to make them grow fast. I raise my own cattle so I am absolutely sure of their origins. I know most of our readers aren't in a position to do this, so I suggest that you look for the purest, most reliable organic source you can find. Then the alkaline-acid ratio will be less pressing.

The dangers of sugar

Let's state it very simply: Sugar feeds cancer. Cancer craves sugar. If you have or have had cancer, sugar is not healthy for you.

If you want to avoid cancer, keep away from the sugar, because an abundance of processed sugar in your diet can cause imbalances in the normal healthy pH balance, moving your body toward a low acid environment that is hospitable to cancer cells.

Here's how sugar works to feed cancer and kill the host if it is not stopped:

If you've ever made wine, you'll know that fermentation requires sugar. In the human body, the metabolism of cancer is approximately eight times greater than the metabolism of normal cells.

So, the cancer has a voracious appetite for sugar. The cancer cells are constantly on the verge of starvation causing the body to run in overdrive trying to feed this hunger, setting up a vicious cycle, helping cancer cells grow and creating more sugar hunger.

When the cancer's food supply, sugar, is cut off, the cancer cells begin to starve unless they can force the body to produce enough sugar to feed them. If the cancer is rapidly growing, you can actually starve the cancer to death by avoiding simple sugars..

We know this sounds grim, but here's the harsh reality: Most cancer patients actually starve to death as the body tries desperately to convert anything it can get, even protein, into sugar to feed the cancer cells. It begins to cannibalize itself, eating muscle tissue, a condition called cachexia.

Knowing this makes it quite apparent why we shouldn't eat a diet high in simple sugars. If you have been diagnosed with cancer or you are at high risk for cancer, you certainly want to avoid all foods high in sugar and simple carbohydrates. If you're trying to

CHAPTER FOUR: BALANCE THROUGH DIET AND LIFESTYLE

prevent cancer (and who isn't?), we suggest you sharply limit your intake of simple sugars. A piece of cake on your birthday is OK. Anything more could be dangerous to your health. But you should even say "No" to that if it is going to make you "fall off of the wagon" and start eating sugar again.

Sugar is truly addicting, just like alcohol. So if you can't eat just one piece – just say "No." One of the most common forms of simple sugar in our food is high fructose corn syrup, found in a wide variety of foods where you might not expect it including juice drinks, ketchup, many processed foods and even some so-called health foods like energy bars.

Healthy fats

What fats are good and which ones are bad?

The absolute best fats come from fatty cold water fish, like salmon and tuna. These healthy fats are called Omega-3 fatty acids and their components have been credited with protecting the heart and cardiovascular system, joints, brain and, most importantly for our purpose, to protect against cancer.

Even more importantly, the components of fish oil have been shown to be particularly effective in preventing hormonally-dependent cancers like breast cancer.

We recommend eating fish once or twice a week and taking a fish oil supplement (1-3 grams) daily.

Other healthy fats: olive oil, a great source of another essential fat called Omega-6, any seed or nut oils, like walnut and sesame and coconut oil, a much-maligned oil that has tremendous health benefits. We know, some of these are acidifying foods, so use them sparingly and in keeping with the balance recommended in the alkaline diet.

Stay away from:

- Any oils that are solid at room temperature (i.e. Crisco-type fats, lard, etc.) except coconut oil;

- Hydrogenated fats and trans fatty acids: fortunately these are now included on labeling, so your job of detecting them is easier. Most commercial baked goods are full of these harmful fats.

- Canola oil: It has the appearance of something healthy. It is made by irradiating rapeseed oil which is not digestible by humans.

KATHLEEN SAYS: Fish oil is my absolute favorite supplement. I can't eat fish, so I am religious about taking fish oil every day.

While I take several supplements, if some strange decree limited me to taking just one, it would be fish oil. I think it's that important for protecting every single system in our bodies.

Water

Water is the stuff of life. Without it, we can only live for a few days.

Drink it, savor it, fill yourself with it. Your body craves it for health.

Water is alkaline, assuming you are drinking high quality water.

Unfortunately, most tap water is junk and after it is chlorinated and passes through a maze of pipes made of a variety of toxic metals, it is no longer healthy.

So.... you buy bottled water? That's not a good choice either. Not only are the billions of empty plastic bottles clogging our landfills, the water is interacting with the carcinogenic phthalates in the plastic water bottles. Remember phthalates from our discussion of early puberty in Chapter 2? Well, those xenoestrogens that affect children affect everyone.

These false estrogens, scientifically known as estrogen receptor stimulants, have been proven to increase the risk of various types of cancer, including breast and prostate cancer. If you need to carry water with you and glass containers are not feasible, make the next best choice by buying a hard plastic container made from polyethylene designated #2HDPE or #4HDPE.

If you're not yet ready to buy a place in the country and get all of your water from a clean, deep well, here's the right choice for your source of water: Install a whole house water filter and rest easy. Yes, this will cost about $1,000 for the average home. It will filter every faucet, including your shower, a much–forgotten source of the chlorine and other chemicals in tap water. Why even filter the shower water? The skin is a very effective way to get chemicals into the body and the hot water opens your pores so your skin is literally "drinking" in the water. The $1,000 cost may seem like a lot, but it is worth it in terms of protecting yourself and your family from toxic chemicals and xenoestrogens. There are some very good water systems that come with ionizers

If you need to save up a bit to buy the whole Magilla, the next best choice is an under-the-sink water filter that will let you have pure drinking water. Third best if the budget simply doesn't allow anything else is one of those inexpensive pitcher-type water filters, although we're not really fond of those because they are made of plastic. If you use one of them, immediately transfer your filtered water to a glass container for storage.

Alcohol

There is conflicting evidence about the benefits of drinking alcoholic beverages and your overall health, but there is some quite specific information about drinking and breast cancer: Several studies suggest women who have more than one drink a day are at an increased risk of breast cancer.

In fact, more than one drink a day can increase the risk of breast cancer by as much as 30 percent in women who are already at high risk for the disease, according to a study of nearly a quarter of a million women sponsored by the American Cancer Society. And Johns Hopkins researchers found that drinking even small amounts can more than double the risk for women who are genetically predisposed to breast cancer.

It's OK to have a glass of wine a day if you're not at high risk (see Chapter 9), but don't start drinking alcohol because it's "healthy." If you're at high risk for breast cancer, give serious consideration to avoiding alcohol altogether.

Manage your weight

There is a growing connection between breast cancer and obesity, especially excess weight in the abdomen and upper body. For example, almost half of all breast cancer cases occur in obese women.

Overweight women are more likely to develop breast cancer because their bodies produce more estrogen than thin women do.

High levels of estrogen stimulate certain types of breast cancer tumors to grow. A study published in the Journal of the National Cancer Institute in 2003, shows that the average concentration of estrogens in obese women was between 50 percent and 219 percent higher than in thin women, and the risk of breast cancer increased from 2 to 18 percent for each 5-point increase in the body mass index (BMI), a measure of weight and height used to determine obesity.

Managing your weight is difficult. Notice we didn't say you should "lose" weight. Think back to the lessons of The Secret™: Losing weight says to your subconscious mind that you are losing a part of yourself. Instead, let yourself be in control and manage your weight.

Simply by subscribing to the alkaline diet, you'll be eating more low-calorie fruits and vegetables and other lower fat, better-for-you foods.

Just by staying away from the acid junk foods, cookies, potato chips, ice cream and candy, you'll most likely be able to get in control of your weight.

And, of course your exercise program will help kick your metabolism into higher gear.

Don't smoke

Smoking is the single most harmful thing we can do to our bodies. You might eat the purest diet imaginable, but if you smoke, you'll be throwing all those good intentions into the trash can.

We are also aware of how difficult it is to break the smoking habit. Some say it is more difficult to get off nicotine than it is to kick a heroin addiction.

Since neither of us has ever smoked, it's easy to say, "Just quit." We won't do that because we've seen the suffering of so many friends and relatives. We've watched those we love die terrible deaths that could have been avoided if they had been able to stop smoking.

Cigarettes are full of proven cancer-causing substances. But their harm goes beyond distributing carcinogens through your body.

Let's think back to Dr. Otto Warburg and his discovery that oxygen-starved cells become cancerous. Now think about what smoking does to your lungs. Right! It coats them with tar, nicotine and other substances that block the free distribution of oxygen to the entire body. So cigarette smoking is a double whammy: cigarette smoking causes cancer and it starves the body of oxygen, promoting the growth of cancer cells.

Smoking is a huge risk factor for developing breast cancer.

A large five-year study published in the Journal of the National Cancer Institute in 2004 yielded these daunting results:

- Women who were still smoking when they filled out the questionnaire were 32 percent more likely to develop breast cancer than those who had never smoked.

- The risk of breast cancer rises significantly with the number of years and the number of cigarettes a woman smokes. The longer they smoke and the more cigarettes they smoke per month, the greater their risk of breast cancer.

- Quitting smoking has almost immediate positive effects. Over time, former smokers are able to reduce their risk to almost the same levels as those who have never smoked.

- Passive smoking does not seem to increase breast cancer risk.

So you've got the message. It's time to stop smoking today. Don't wait until tomorrow. Don't procrastinate.

But how you ask? We say, "Use any method that works for you." Patches, nicotine gums, hypnosis, homeopathics. There are many tools on the market and, while the results are individual, they all work.

The techniques taught in *The Secret*™ and in *The Healing Codes*™ can be immensely effective in helping you stop smoking.

In fact, smoking is such a health destroyer that you might decide to make a trade off: Put a somewhat toxic substance like Wellbutrin (a prescription drug well-researched to help people stop smoking) in your body to ride yourself of a destructive habit. If that's what it takes, go ahead and do it. We know, that's a big leap for the two of us who are so steeped in finding natural means to address health problems. However, smoking is so serious and so destructive that we even recommend a pharmaceutical if that's what it takes to get cigarettes out of your life.

The key to successfully quitting smoking is that you must really want to quit. Without a deep commitment, nothing will be effective.

Chapter 5

THERMOGRAMS, YES, MAMMOGRAMS, NO!

Doctors and the medical community have pounded this into our heads throughout our reproductive lives: You need an annual mammogram from the time you are 40 on, they'll tell you. For more than two decades, these painful annual screenings have become a way of life for millions of women.

They'll tell you mammograms can reduce your chances of dying from breast cancer by about 30 percent by helping detect early stage breast cancers too small for your monthly BSE to detect.

What your doctor won't tell you is that there is no evidence that screening for breast cancer with mammograms saves women's lives. It is interesting to note that although mammography does lead to the discovery of smaller, earlier-stage cancerous tumors, it still does not improve breast cancer survival rates any more than physical examination alone!

What your doctor won't tell you is that a mammogram exposes you to approximately 1,000 times the amount of radiation you'd get in a chest X-ray. If that's not enough, the radiation is stored in your cells and so it accumulates to significant levels over time if you're getting an annual mammogram.

What your doctor won't tell you is that the extreme compression of your breast tissues in a mammography machine can damage delicate breast tissue and may even break open cancerous tumors and send them throughout your breast where they will grow and spread.

DR. BEN SAYS: You may have seen claims that mammograms find many small cancers. What you aren't told is that these small cancers are actually a type of cancer called DCIS (ductal carcinoma in situ) that rarely kills anyone. In fact, many pathologists don't even call it cancer.

In fact, if you were to be able to check the breast tissue of every woman over 60, you'd find DCIS cells present in almost every one. These cells are living happily there without causing any problems.

That is, of course, unless you were to squeeze the breast repeatedly between two pieces of plastic and x-ray them, maybe popping them out of the duct where the cells can travel through the lymphatics to the bones or liver. I have seen two of these cases of metastatic ductal breast cancer without any cancer in the breast at all. Both of these ladies were faithful mammography clients.

European experts who reviewed the health benefits of mammograms were unable to find any evidence at all for their benefit all the way back in 2001, undermining the findings of the initial study on which modern mammograms are justified.

And the nation's largest medical specialty group, the American College of Physicians, recently issued new guidelines questioning the wisdom of having mammograms, particularly for women between 40 and 50. The 120,000-member association that represents internists, said the risks of mammography may outweigh its benefits.

Another recent study found that a costly computerized system to help read mammograms was no better at finding cancer than traditional mammography and led to many more false alarms. The computerized systems are used in some 30 percent of all mammography centers, where they are driving up costs with no clear benefit. Government and private insurers have been urged to reconsider whether the systems are worth covering.

And finally, the National Cancer Institute admits that monthly breast self-examinations (BSEs) following a brief training, in conjunction with annual clinical breast examinations (CBEs) by a trained health care professional, are at least as effective as mammography.

Want more evidence? An article published in the Journal of the National Cancer Institute nearly seven years ago said that the more mammograms a woman has had, the greater the chance she will get a result known in medical terms as a "false positive." That means that the radiologist who reads the mammogram sees a suspicious change in the breast tissue.

False positives, which ultimately turn out to be benign or noncancerous, usually end up with a woman having further testing, including biopsies and even needless lumpectomies and mastectomies. This doesn't factor in the incredible stress that comes with these false positives and the unnecessary procedures that can accompany them. The study of patients at Harvard hospitals in 2000 reported that if a woman has had 10 mammograms, there is a 50 percent chance she will get a false positive. Worse yet, women with high risk factors for breast cancer had a 100 percent false positive rate. That means every single one had at least one breast cancer scare that turned out to be baseless.

The American Cancer Society guidelines recommend all women over age 40 have a screening mammogram every year, so by the time a woman reaches age 50, she would have had nine mammograms and quite likely at least one false positive.

We have many concerns about these tests, but perhaps none so great as the stress that results from a false positive that may in itself create a disease condition, possibly even breast cancer.

You may have been in this position yourself: You have a mammogram and you wait for the results. After a few days, you get a call that your doctor wants you to return for a "diagnostic mammogram" or an ultrasound. What runs through your head? It's perfectly natural to become preoccupied with the idea that you might have breast cancer. Day and night until the ordeal is over, you're thinking "Oh my God, do I have breast cancer?" You lose sleep. You become massively stressed and fearful.

From the principles of *The Secret*™ and *The Healing Codes*™ we've taught you about the Law of Attraction and the role of stress in causing the disease process, you know that this is setting you up for something bad.

We think that mammograms are a terrible and needless burden placed on women that may be unwittingly causing the very disease they are intended to detect and treat early.

We think mammograms are highly detrimental to your body, mind and spirit. We recommend that you avoid them as a screening tool. There is a time when they are appropriate as a cancer detection device, but we now have MRIs, which we will talk about later.

Fortunately, there is a safe and effective alternative to mammography.

DR. BEN SAYS: Mammograms should never be used as a preventive tool because they are so potentially damaging.

I'm not even a big fan of using mammograms to diagnose something suspicious because of the high number of false positives, the exposure to radiation and the compression that can actually squeeze cancer cells out and into the lymphatic system. We have alternatives that work much better than mammograms and that can help a woman and her doctor know more about her breasts and keep them healthy.

Thermography is absolutely the best preventive tool because it can pick up a potential problem long before a mammogram might.

Thermograms for health

Thermograms are every woman's best option for healthy breasts. They offer a noninvasive, painless and safe way of tracking a woman's breast health over a period of years. If it matters to you, thermography is FDA approved and can be used for all types of body tissue, not breasts alone. A thermogram offers information about your breasts that no other technology can provide. Its best use is as a preventive tool to track a woman's breast health over a period of years and to catch potential problems before they become big problems.

Thermograms are not new. They've been around for more than 30 years, although the newest generation of the technology is far more reliable and effective than earlier systems.

Thermography is an infrared heat digital imaging system. It uses no radiation, is painless, noninvasive and the machine does not even touch your skin. It shows color images of heat in the tissue and gray scale, which shows vascularity or circulation in the breast.

How it works

A thermogram is made by a specialized type of digital camera that captures an image of the circulation of blood in your tissues. Having a thermogram is as easy as having your picture taken.

Normal tissue has a blood supply that is under the control of the autonomic nervous system (ANS). The ANS can either increase or decrease blood flow to cells. Abnormal (cancerous and pre-cancerous) tissue, on the other hand, ensures its own survival by secreting chemicals that override this ANS regulation, thereby ensuring its own steady blood supply. Cancer can be thought of as being "off the power grid" of the body.

When your hands are placed in cold water, an ANS reflex occurs in the breasts. Generally speaking, this reflex causes the blood vessels in non-cancerous tissue to constrict, but does not result in constriction of blood vessels supplying cancerous tissues. The resulting difference in blood flow can result in cancer showing up as "hot spots" on thermograms.

By measuring the temperature of many different points on the skin before and after the cold stimulus, a thermogram monitors changes in circulation that can signal the presence of a tumor. The actual temperature, as well as how it changes in response to the cold stimulus, provides information about the function of the breast tissues that correspond to the points being measured.

A thermogram is an early warning system to tell you that you may be headed for trouble. This gives you ample opportunity to change your diet and your lifestyle, and, most importantly, to change the way you are thinking and not fall into fear and panic that will imbed new and powerful cellular memories that will further compromise your immune system and impair your body's ability to fight off the cancerous invader.

Breast thermography does not diagnose breast cancer. Instead, it detects changes in breast tissue that indicate the presence of cancer or pre-cancerous states. Breast cancer is diagnosed in a number of ways that we'll discuss at length in Chapter 10.

Breast thermography has several unique abilities that make it well worth your while:

- It can give tumor warning signals far in advance, up to ten years ahead of the occurrence of invasive tumor growth.

- Unlike after-the-fact warning when a tumor is already present like you'd get with a mammogram, ultrasound, MRI or CT scan, thermography can assess a woman's risk of developing a tumor and can also assess her hormonal status.

- It can also distinguish between fibrocystic breasts and cancerous tumors.

- It can examine breasts with implants, which cannot be adequately screened with routine mammography because the compression could damage the implant and because the implant can actually block the view of deeper parts of the breast.

- It is effective for breasts of all sizes. Women with very small or very large breasts often do not receive adequate images from mammograms.

- Young women with dense breasts may not receive adequate imaging.

- The rate of false negatives and false positives is less than 10 percent, much better than for mammograms.

Women with a family history of breast cancer are at greater risk of developing the disease, but 75 percent of women who get breast cancer have no family history of the disease. Regardless of your family history, if your thermogram is abnormal, you run a future risk of breast cancer that is 10 times higher than someone with a first degree relative (mother, sister or daughter) with the disease. Thermography is the only technology to provide women with a future risk assessment.

If a thermogram shows a woman is at risk of developing breast cancer, this can be a warning she needs to work to improve her breast health. Monitoring with regular check-ups and thermography will show improvements with time or possibly the earliest signs that a problem may exist. This information lets a woman and her doctor know when or if there is a risk of a problem developing and measures like those we discuss in this book can be taken to prevent a tumor from growing and spreading.

Since one of the greatest risk factors for the development of breast cancer is total lifetime exposure to estrogen, normalizing the balance of the hormones in the breast may be the first and most significant step in prevention. Breast thermography is the only known non-invasive procedure that can detect estrogen dominance in the breasts. If a woman's thermographic images suggest a relative progesterone deficiency (estrogen dominance), treatment of this condition may play an important role in prevention. (For more on estrogen dominance, perimenopause and menopause, see Chapter 6.)

With treatment from her doctor, a woman can use this information to balance the hormones in her breasts. Follow-up thermograms are compared to the baseline estrogen dominant images as part of the treatment monitoring process.

All women can benefit from thermography, but those between the ages of 30 and 50 have the best results because their breast tissues are denser than those of older women and therefore other screening methods can be less exact.

Preparing for a thermogram

1. Avoid natural or artificial tanning for one week prior to your thermogram.

2. Refrain from saunas, steam baths, and hot or cold packs for at least 24 hours prior to your thermogram. Do not bathe, shower, or exercise during the hour prior to your thermogram appointment. Wait for 36 hours after a high fever before having a thermogram.

3. Refrain from using any tobacco products and consuming any caffeine including caffeinated coffee, tea, or sodas for two hours prior to your thermogram.

4. Remove large jewelry prior to imaging; however, small necklaces actually enable the thermogram technician to sharpen the focus of your thermogram.

5. Avoid shaving your underarms or applying any underarm deodorants or antiperspirants in addition to all powders, creams, or lotions on your arms or chest on the day of your thermogram.

6. Avoid any physical exam or compression of your breasts including self-examination of the breasts, mammography, or ultrasound of the breast for at least 24 hours prior to your scheduled breast thermogram.

7. Wait three months after breast surgery or completion of chemotherapy and/or radiation before having a thermogram.

8. Do not exercise, or engage in any activities that will increase your blood pressure the day of the exam.

9. Do not smoke or drink alcohol for a minimum of 24 hours before your appointment.

10. Take only medications that you take regularly. Your physician can give you further information.

11. Wear comfortable clothing that covers your arms and make sure to wear socks. A loose button-down shirt is great.

12. Do not wear tight clothing, including belts. Anything that leaves a red mark when you remove it is too tight.

13. Avoid confrontation or emotional stress on the day of your thermogram. That can quite literally raise your skin temperature.

What happens during an exam?

When you arrive at your appointment, you'll be asked to take off all clothing and jewelry above the waist.

Then you'll be asked to wait in an environmentally controlled room for about 15 minutes. This will get your skin temperature to a definable level.

When you are brought into the imaging room, you'll be standing in front of the camera with your fingers clasped behind your head, elbows pointing out to the sides. Between 7 and 9 views of your breast will be taken, depending on the size of your breasts.

A second set of images is often taken after your hands have been submerged in cold water for one minute. Some thermographers do not use this technique, and that is just fine.

Results

Your thermogram will be read by a licensed thermologist and, usually, by your doctor as well. Breast thermograms receive one of five ratings that range from TH1 (no detectable thermal abnormalities) to TH5 (detection of thermal abnormalities correlating with very significant risk for breast cancer). Any positive result signals a need for further evaluation. Early thermal abnormalities may result in a recommendation to repeat thermography for comparison in 60 to 120 days. Depending on the thermology rating and other forms of evaluation, a referral may be made for targeted ultrasound or to a breast specialist.

Doctors trained in holistic medicine may also recommend nutritional, metabolic, environmental, or lifestyle interventions to address early thermal abnormalities.

Finding a thermogram provider

For more information on thermography and to find a thermography center near you, go to www.thermographytest.com

Cost of a thermogram

The cost of a thermogram is reasonable, generally between $100 and $200, depending on where you live.

Many insurance companies will cover thermography, but since there seems to be an endless variety of insurance plans, be sure to check with your insurer and the provider of the thermogram.

If your insurance plan includes "out-of-network" and non standard-of-care benefits, you will probably receive some insurance reimbursement. Your insurance company may require a referral from your doctor or pre-approval or authorization. For your doctor's information, the billing code (known as a CPT code) is 93762. Knowing this number will help you get reimbursement.

But what if your insurance doesn't cover it? Well, we think your breasts are worth it! We hope you do, too.

If you're at high risk

We'll be talking about your risk factors in Chapter 8, so if you're unsure if you are high risk, you might want to skip to that chapter now while you're considering what type of screening you need.

If you are at high risk for breast cancer (biggest risk: breast cancer in your mother or sister and, if you know, the presence of the BRCA1 or BRCA2 genes) or if you underwent radiation therapy of the chest, your doctor and your insurance company may agree that an annual MRI screening is warranted. An estimated 1.4 million American women fall into this category, but that doesn't mean their health insurance companies will automatically cover the $1,500-$4,000 cost of an MRI. Prepare for at least a minor skirmish, if not a major battle, to get an MRI if you and your doctor think it is necessary.

Some ammo for your battle: Guidelines just issued by the American Cancer Society recommend annual MRI scans in addition to mammograms for all women at high risk of developing breast cancer, starting at age 30.

One new study found that MRI scans could find tumors that mammograms had missed in a small percentage of women. The downside is that the scans are so sensitive they pick up lots of suspicious but harmless growths. These false positives cause anxiety on the part of the patient, they are expensive and they may prompt doctors to initiate unnecessary treatments.

All of that said, MRIs may find cancer invisible to other screening and diagnostic methods.

Dr. Ben recommends discussing the upside and the downside of MRIs with your doctor and your insurance company if your risk is high, but to couple them with thermograms rather than mammograms.

Chapter 6 HORMONES, PERIMENOPAUSE AND MENOPAUSE, OH MY!

Hormones play a major role in everyone's life, and derogatory hormone jokes about women notwithstanding, both sexes are often unaware of hormonal ebbs and flows until they catch up with us with a vengeance somewhere about the time middle age hits.

There comes a time in every woman's life when levels of sex hormones start to yo-yo and our reproductive lives draw to a close.

Before you panic, let us assure you that your life is far from over. In fact, the best part may be just beginning, with a newfound freedom that usually comes from more time for yourself, fewer or no children around the house and a new sense of self-worth. In fact, we are far more fortunate than our ancestors in that our expanded lifespan means the majority of women still have one-third of their lives to live after menopause, not to mention the freedom of not having to put up with a monthly period ever again!

Perimenopause: the change before 'The Change'

Perimenopause (the years before menopause) and menopause itself signal a new time in a woman's life when she can do as she likes without so many responsibilities to a growing family.

Our hormonal clocks tick every moment of our lives. It's just when perimenopause and menopause hit, that the clock sometimes runs fast and sometimes runs slow.

Let's start with some basic biology that will help you understand what is happening at this stage of your life.

Through a woman's life, her pituitary gland sends signals to her ovaries to produce estrogen. Sometimes the ovaries respond to those messages, and sometimes, as she gets older, the ovaries ignore the message.

Perimenopause is the time of life when those messages start to be ignored on a regular basis. They're a lot like those insistent messages on your answering machine that you just don't feel like returning.

Perimenopause can start as early as a woman's mid-30s, but more typically, perimenopause begins in the late 40s. Those fluctuating estrogen and progesterone levels cause a variety of symptoms, most of them simply annoying, but some can be serious. A wide array of symptoms can accompany perimenopause, but the most common are hot flashes, mood swings and irritability, loss of short term memory, insomnia, night sweats, loss of hair and depression.

Each woman's perimenopause is different, and some barely notice the change while others suffer greatly. Most women fall somewhere in the middle and experience a couple of symptoms that are particularly bothersome.

That's the key: The symptoms of perimenopause are usually bothersome or annoying. Occasionally, they have profound effects on a woman's quality of life, but perimenopause rarely produces any symptoms that are life threatening.

However, the long-term effects of declining hormones and the long years of menopause can produce some serious health problems, increasing the risk of hormone-related breast, ovarian, cervical and endometrial cancers, heart disease, stroke, osteoporosis and Alzheimer's disease.

It's not just the estrogen

Many women, and sadly, too many doctors, believe that perimenopause is a matter of nose-diving estrogen production.

Actually, one of the first clinical signs of approaching menopause is declining progesterone level.

At the same time, estrogen levels may remain stable or even increase.

To further complicate matters, estrogen is actually a name for a group of several hormones, any of which can become unbalanced.

Progesterone and estrogen play a delicate dance of balance throughout your menstrual cycle, rising and falling as the cycle progresses.

- Estrogen promotes the growth of the uterine lining, the endometrium, to nourish a fetus. Progesterone keeps those endometrial cells from growing too rapidly.

- Estrogen slows the production of thyroid hormones and progesterone speeds it up.

- Estrogen increases salt and fluid retention and progesterone helps rid your body of excess fluids.

Estrogen dominance

Without sufficient progesterone, as typically takes place in peri-menopause, estrogen becomes dominant, not because there is too little estrogen, but because there is too much estrogen circulating through the system with insufficient amounts of progesterone to balance it out. When all those estrogen molecules start partying around in the body with no progesterone to act as a dance partner, it can mean trouble.

In addition, we have those xenoestrogens or toxic environmental estrogens we talked about in Chapter 2 that play havoc with hormone balance. These estrogens are generated by plastics, pesticides and toxic chemicals in the environment and in the hormones injected into dairy cows and animals slaughtered for food. Or they may come into your body through a well meaning physician who has given you hormone replacement therapy with equine derived hormones. When these unnatural estrogen molecules get into our bodies, they try to act like natural estrogen molecules. When they bind to the hormone receptor sites, they increase the risk of rapid cell division.

The free estrogen molecules and the toxic xenoestrogen molecules cycle around the body looking for a home. When they find an estrogen receptor site, it's like the hormone molecule is a key and the receptor on the cell is a lock. The hormone molecule opens that lock and moves right on in, sometimes to perform its proper function, and sometimes not.

When the estrogen molecules find their way into breast cancer cells, the estrogen feeds them, nourishes them and encourages them to reproduce. It keeps them "turned on" and active rather than living their natural life spans and dying when they are supposed to. These cells actually become almost immortal, at least until they kill their host.

Conventional hormone replacement

Now that we've examined the delicate dance of the hormones, you can well imagine that these strange hormones and hormones in wrong proportions for humans can be problematic.

Most conventional doctors will tell their patients that perimeno-pause and menopause signal a shortfall of estrogen. This couldn't be farther from the truth and there is tons of scientific research to back it up. These doctors just aren't paying attention!

Conventional doctors' solution for this so-called "shortage" of estrogen is to give you more estrogen. From what you've learned in this chapter alone, you know that can be dangerous.

But it gets worse. Not only does your doctor want you to have more estrogen, despite some very sobering research, conventional doctors are still pressing women to take hormone replacement therapy (HRT) made from the urine of pregnant mares. These unnatural estrogens and synthetic progesterone are prescribed under the guise that this horse estrogen will protect them from heart disease, strokes, osteoporosis and even breast cancer. Equine-based HRT actually increases the risk of all these diseases in a frightening way.

Bear with us now. We know it's getting a little complicated, but we're making a crucial point here.

Estradiol, the type of estrogen believed to be the most carcinogenic of the human estrogen trio, is particularly attracted to those hormone receptor sites.

Estradiol is present in high proportions in many synthetic types of hormone replacement, although only in small amounts in Pre-marin™, the popular horse-urine based hormone replacement. Instead, Premarin™ (PREgnant MAres' uRINe) contains four to eight times the amount of estrone, one of the three major forms of estrogen found in humans, and no estriol, the most abundant type of estrogen in humans and the least problematic. Premarin™ also contains equilin, a horse estrogen not found in humans. In simple terms: Horse es-trogen looks nothing like human estrogen. There are at least 23 types of estrogen in equine estrogen only one of which is common to hu-mans. This type of "therapy" will make an old nag out of you – pun intended!

Yet, since 1942, when the synthetic hormone replacement drug Premarin™ came on the market, conventional doctors have touted it as the best thing that ever happened to menopausal women. They are not to be blamed for believing what the drug companies told them. We know, it's hard to abandon "conventional wisdom," but the truth turned out to be 180 degrees from the promise.

In the summer of 2002, the Women's Health Initiative, a large scientific study sponsored by the National Institutes of Health, was stopped after preliminary results showed women taking Prempro™ (Premarin™ plus Progest™, a synthetic drug meant to be like progesterone) had no protection against disease, as women had been promised for 60 years.

Instead, women who took the drug were found to have a dramatically increased risk of serious and potentially fatal diseases.

Myths about heart protection were busted wide open when results showed that the women taking the combination actually had 27 percent more heart attacks than those who got the placebo.

They had a 26 percent higher risk of breast cancer (this wasn't really a surprise), but the increased risk of invasive breast cancer led the National Institutes of Health to stop the study because of the alarming risk to participants.

That's not to speak of 38 percent more strokes and more than double the number of blood clots.

A year later, researchers found that women taking Prempro™ had twice the risk of dementia, the clinical term for Alzheimer's and a variety of other diseases of mental deterioration.

It's not nice to fool Mother Nature. Women aren't horses and their hormonal makeup is vastly different. While horse urine may be effective at easing some of the more unpleasant symptoms of menopause, the science is now solid: It dramatically increases your risk of serious disease. In three words: Don't take it!

Bioidentical hormone replacement

Here's where the trumpets blare and the brass bands march down the street: Bioidentical hormones.

These are natural ways to safely duplicate these hormones exactly as your body manufactured them in its prime.

Your doctor probably won't mention this to you because it's likely he or she doesn't know about these natural hormones that have been available for more than 20 years.

You can get natural hormones only by prescription, and their manufacture is regulated by the FDA. They are backed by clinical research and they are safe.

Bioidentical hormones are made from highly purified chemicals originally derived from soy and wild yams, but there is a complex manufacturing process that transforms them into a carbon copy of the hormones you had at the peak of your hormone production. They're not plant or herbal extracts. They're called natural because of the origin of their chemical structure.

Bioidentical hormones are keys that fit exactly into hormone receptor locks, while synthetic ones don't fit exactly and some can stay too long or not long enough, increasing your long-term risks or worse.

Bioidentical hormones are not usually given in a standardized, one-size-fits-all dose, but tailored to a woman's individual hormone test results. They are generally given at low doses, because chemically their makeup is identical to natural estrogen.

Best of all, as far as anyone knows, there is no increased risk of hormone-related cancers, heart disease, osteoporosis or dementia with bioidentical hormones.

Finding a doctor

First, you'll need to find a doctor who knows about natural hormone replacement or who is willing to learn. This isn't easy.

In these days of managed care, your doctor is likely to be more pressured and less informed than at any time in the last century.

You're incredibly lucky if you have a doctor who is already up to date on natural hormone replacement and is willing to conduct the necessary testing, customized prescription and monitoring of your hormonal state.

If you don't know such a doctor and haven't found one, you'll need to become an educator for your doctor. Prepare for the possibility you may meet with resistance, even in the wake of the Women's Health Initiative. Many doctors will still insist that equine-estrogens and progestin are the standard and they should be good enough for you. They're neither the standard nor are they good enough for you.

Here's what to do:

- Schedule an appointment with your doctor and discuss what you've learned about natural hormone replacement.

- Tell your doctor your symptoms in simple terms. It helps to have your list in writing so you don't skip over anything.

- Express your wish to use bioidentical hormones.

- Go to that appointment forearmed with information.

- Ask for your dosages to be individualized. If your doctor does not know how to do this, many compounding pharmacies are willing to assist in determining your precise needs.

- Ask for your hormone levels to be monitored on an ongoing basis, at least once a year.

Meeting resistance

Let your doctor know that many major pharmaceutical companies are now producing bioidentical hormones, among them the estrogens Estrace™, Climara™, Vivelle™ and Estraderm™ and progesterone's Prometrium™ and Crinone™. You've made some headway if your doctor wants to prescribe one of these for you—but while they're bioidentical to a hypothetical 35-year old woman, they aren't customized to you. You'd do better with a customized formula designed exclusively for you.

Most doctors are reasonable folks, and they are open to learning something new. If your doctor is neither reasonable nor open to new information, you might want to give serious consideration to finding a doctor who is.

The next step: compounding pharmacy

Next, you'll need a pharmacist who specializes in compounding (making prescriptions by hand) and titrating (individualizing the dosage).

Don't look for this at your local CVS or Walgreen's. They'll look at you like you just flew in from Mars (or Venus)! You're best off if you can find a compounding pharmacy that specializes in women's health and hormone therapy. In fact this is the easy way to find a physician who will prescribe bioidentical hormones. They will know which doctors are familiar with them and know how to prescribe them.

To find a compounding pharmacy, go to the International Academy of Compounding Pharmacists website: www.iacprx.org or phone them at (800) 927-4227, ext. 30.

You may have to do some additional footwork to find one that specializes in hormone therapy, but this will give you a good start.

Many compounding pharmacies will work directly with your doctor and send prescriptions by mail, so it isn't essential that the pharmacy be located close to you.

Insurance obstacles

Congratulations! You've gotten this far, but you've got one last obstacle to overcome: Your insurance company. You may have already stumbled a little on this one. Many insurance companies balk at hormone testing, especially if your doctor prefers saliva testing. You may have to pay for your prescriptions yourself.

Saliva testing typically costs $60-$150 once a year and prescriptions for your natural hormones will run in the neighborhood of $50 a month.

You may get some help if your doctor will write a letter of medical necessity to your insurance company, explaining that the care you need is not available within the existing scope of your health care plan. You may need to write a letter to your insurance company yourself, and become an advocate and an educator again.

Good luck!

Chapter 7 # THE HEALING CODES: DON'T LET STRESS RUN YOUR LIFE

Stress is the major bugaboo of modern life. It is the wild dog snapping at our heels, keeping us running from the moment our eyes open on a new day until we fall exhausted into bed at night. It is the monster that lives under our beds, stalking us even as we sleep, walking in our dreams and snapping us into sudden awakening long before the alarm sounds.

Science tells us that 85 percent of all illness is caused by stress. While that is a startling number, Dr. Ben thinks that, on the physiological level, stress is the underlying cause of nearly 100 percent of all illness.

So what is stress?

It's that itchy fidgety feeling you get when you're late for work and you can't find your keys and the dog has peed on the floor and your firstborn decides now is the time to recite for you the entire plot of the latest kiddie book he's read.

It's that vague feeling of disquiet when in a solitary moment you can't for the life of you recall what important thing you forgot.

It's getting into bed exhausted and finding your mind insists on re-runs of your day (or worse yet, last week or last month), who said what and who didn't say what, where you'll find the money to pay the mortgage, followed by an endless repetition of your to-do list.

Stress is also what happens when a mother sees a tree fall on her child and, with superhuman strength she lifts the tree and tosses it to the side like a matchstick.

Stress is what happens when you encounter a mountain lion while you're hiking on a lonely mountain trail and you need to make a decision whether to run (bad idea in this case) or fight (not really a good idea, either) or stay perfectly still and hope it goes away.

The anatomy of stress

If you can imagine the last two scenarios above, you're probably already getting a sense of the physical responses your body would make to a genuine threat. Your heart starts to pound. Your muscles tense. Your mouth becomes dry. Your thought processes are fiercely focused on only one thing: Survival.

You probably wouldn't be as aware of it, but other things are happening to help your physical body survive at all costs:

- More blood is pumping to your muscles to help you be stronger and faster;
- Your adrenal glands start pumping out adrenaline to fuel the process;
- Your body's energy reserves have been diverted from non-essential functions like digestion and immune system function so all your resources are directed toward survival;
- Your blood pressure is increasing;
- Your breathing becomes more rapid;
- Your body begins drawing on all the possible glucose stores it has, from the liver, muscles, from food sources and even from protein to provide the energy necessary to keep you going;
- You begin to sweat profusely, cooling those overheated muscles so they can continue to do what you need them to do.
- Your immune system is completely shut down.

We are hard-wired for survival. Stress is a survival mechanism built into our bodies. When we think we are in danger, we instinctively kick into "fight-or-flight" mode. This means our bodies are prepared to fight to the death for survival or to run away from the danger as fast as we can.

The stress response was meant to serve us for survival for a very short period of time, minutes, perhaps an hour or so at most.

Think how dangerous it would be to keep your body in this state of hyperactivity and hyperalertness day after day rather than for a few minutes. Yet most of us do exactly that, burning the candle at both ends, constantly barraged with media messages and keeping ourselves in a state of chronic stress known as toxic stress.

That protection mechanism doesn't serve us very well today when the danger is far more often mental and emotional rather than physical. After all, you can't really fight or run away from a cranky boss, a sick child or the driver who cut you off in traffic. Your body doesn't know you aren't being confronted by a mountain lion, so it starts cranking out adrenaline and glucose and pumping your heart like crazy and taking blood flow away from nonessential functions.

Our bodies can't take it. In response to the chronic state of stress in which most of us find ourselves, our bodies try to compensate for those unrealistic long-term demands by pumping out cortisol to shore up energy levels and ensure survival in any way we can.

We end up with chronic inflammation that increases the risk of heart disease, cancer, osteoporosis and degenerative arthritis; elevated blood sugars that increase the risk of diabetes and its myriad side effects and weight gain and its associated risks, to mention a few.

Researchers have recently identified a unique stress pattern among women they call "tend and befriend." The theory is that women under stress are primarily concerned with tending and protecting their young and forming alliances with a larger group of women for comfort and protection. This new paradigm, almost exclusively the domain of women, somewhat neutralizes the fight-or-flight response. It may be an intuitive response to the toxic stress response, but it can also lead to a chronic stress situation Kathleen likes to call the martyr complex, in which women think they have to take care of everyone, have a career, keep house, keep fit, volunteer, garden, and on and on and on.

Another element of stress

To the toxic stress response, we're going to add cellular memory. This is another element of stress that is only just beginning to be recognized by the scientific community.

To put it in the simplest possible terms: Your body, down to the individual cells, remembers and believes messages about you from throughout your life that may not be true.

These messages are untruths about you and your relationship to your world. Somewhere along the line, you might have been told you were stupid, ugly, not good enough, a loser. These messages may have come from your family, from society, even from generations past. It could have been something said or not said; done or not done.

These messages become more than memories stored in your brain. They become memories stored in each of the trillions of individual cells in your body, each one endlessly repeating the message:

- "You are stupid."
- "You'll never be good enough."
- "You're a loser."
- "You'll always be poor. You'll never have enough."
- "You're ugly."
- "No one cares about you."

You can probably add some of your own to the list.

These lies have literally imbedded themselves into your cells. Then what happens?

Alex Loyd, N.D., PhD, Dr. Ben's partner in *The Healing Codes*™, describes it like this:

> That lie reverberates through the cells in the form of cellular memory. We know the memory is stored in cells all over the body and those cells resonate the lie to other cells. The cells eventually resonate it to the hypothalamus, the part of the brain that plays a key role in the function of the immune system. The hypothalamus then throws a stress switch on the basis of these lies, stressing the immune system. Based on the stress response to these lies, Dr. Ben's Weak Link Theory kicks in and something breaks. It may open the door to cancer, heart disease or any number of diseases, wherever your weak link is.

These imbedded lies are ruling your life. The best medicine and the best science in the world won't heal you until those lies have been converted to positive beliefs about your self-worth and your place in the world. You can say a new truth as many times as you like in an effort to eradicate the old lies, but until you can find a way to imbed a new and true statement into your cellular memory, the stress and the disease resulting from the old lies will continue.

Lack of self-worth

Many women carry cellular memories of unworthiness. A person without a healthy sense of self-worth is always in a place of self-protection. People with low self-worth get a skewed notion that starting to believe the truth about their own goodness and value is somehow threatening. In fact, says Dr. Loyd, the truth is the opposite: Hanging on to an unworthiness issue may be the most threatening thing to your existence. It goes against that survival instinct.

Here's a chain of events that might help you understand how the cellular memory disrupts your entire being, causing you to live in self-destructive and self-sabotaging ways:

- Wrong beliefs about ourselves and our place in the world cause most of the problems we have in life.

- Wrong beliefs are destructive interpretations of internal images.

- Wrong beliefs motivate thoughts, feelings and harmful actions that cause pain to us and to those around us.

- Wrong beliefs cause us to misinterpret our current circumstances as threatening.

- Wrongly perceiving our circumstance as threatening causes stress and shifts our nervous systems into fight-or-flight mode.

Sometimes our interpretations of events that create cellular memories are flawed. Something that happened to you when you were five years old might seem much different to your adult mind, but you still have the lie interpreted by the five-year old encoded in your cells. It is not only unhelpful but it's actually sabotaging your relationships and your health.

Here's a great example:

It's the story of a woman who felt like her entire life had been negatively affected by her relationship with her mother. The main picture she kept remembering was something that happened when she was five years old and her mother gave her sister a popsicle but would not give her one. Her mother had even said at the time, "Your sister has already had lunch. When you have lunch, you can have a popsicle, too."

Remember, this picture of her relationship with her mother was formed with the mind, feelings and intellect of a five-year old. At five, she had interpreted her mother's actions as meaning her mother did not love her as much as she loved her sister. If that was true, there was something wrong with her, and if that was true, others would probably not love her either. It doesn't seem to make sense in terms of rational adult thinking that her problems could stem from this event, but they did!

It's easy to see how almost every individual alive might suffer from this type of misinterpretation that becomes imprinted on cellular memory.

Can you see how such a seemingly innocuous situation can have long ranging effects on your life?

And can you see how shifting those wrong beliefs can change your life for the better in a hurry?

You might not even need to know or remember the specifics of the incidents that a child's mind interpreted wrongly to create these memories. You can simply ask for them to be gone.

Forgiveness

Dr. Ben says he has never seen a cancer that didn't have an underlying issue of lack of forgiveness to it. Dr. Loyd thinks that virtually every type of sickness is rooted in an inability to forgive others or one's self for perceived wrongs.

Forgiveness is a hard thing to find and an even harder thing to make stick. Until you can find a way to forgive others, and more importantly yourself, anger and suspicion will imbed themselves in your cellular memory.

DR. BEN SAYS: Forgiveness is a huge element in the way our lives become disrupted and cellular memories are formed.

Most everyone who has had a Christian upbringing has said The Lord's Prayer at one time or another. What many people don't realize is that a part of The Lord's Prayer is a request for God to forgive us to the same degree we forgive other people.

When we say, "Forgive us our trespasses as just as we forgive those who trespass against us," we are asking not to be forgiven until we forgive our brothers and sisters.

It's the only part of The Lord's Prayer where Jesus goes back and reiterates to make sure we have it crystal clear: If you do not forgive your brothers and sisters here on Earth, your Heavenly Father will not forgive you.

A bit later, a man comes to Jesus and asks how many times he must forgive his brother and Jesus replies, "seven times seventy." By that Jesus means an infinite number of times.

Whether or not The Lord's Prayer fits into your spiritual belief system, the idea of forgiving others so that you can be forgiven is an important element of your healing.

> **THE LORD'S PRAYER**
>
> Our Father, in heaven, hallowed be your name, your kingdom come, your will be done, on earth as it is in heaven. Give us today our daily bread. Forgive us our debts, as we also have forgiven our debtors. And lead us not into temptation, but deliver us from the evil one. Matthew 6: 9-13
>
> (New International Version)

Who is forgiveness really for?

Consider this example: Imagine something really bad happened to you. Imagine you were raped by someone unknown. We can't imagine anything worse or anything more unforgivable. It is terrible and undoubtedly you grapple with thoughts of rage and outrage, violation of your core self and bitterness.

We ask you again: Who is forgiveness really for?

Will all your hate, anger and bitterness hurt the rapist for one minute, even for one second? No. It only hurts you. If you haven't forgiven someone for a wrong done to you, you are bound to that person.

Kathleen has always remembered a sign she saw in the front yard of a little country church that said, "That which angers you controls you."

Forgiveness is for you and you alone. It sets you free.

Holding on to past hurts is like swimming in a rapid current with a cinder block tied to your waist. No matter how skilled a swimmer you are, that cinder block will drag you to the bottom and drown you. Forgiveness cuts the rope and frees you from the burden of that hate, anger and bitterness.

KATHLEEN SAYS: I'm a believer in a just Universe. Whatever you choose to call it, I believe there is retribution for wrong deeds. If someone has perpetrated something unforgivable on you, you can forgive and move on with your own life. You can rest assured that justice will be served in one way or another, in this life or the next.

It's easy to say you forgive someone for a wrong done, but it's easier said than done. It's much harder to keep on forgiving the offender over and over again, day after day, when the old pattern of anger and betrayal re-appears and you think of the situation and you still feel anger.

Dr. Ben tells people in a religious context that forgiveness requires them to be like Jesus: He will forgive us time after time and you're going to have to forgive others time after time. It's an issue that will keep coming back even when you think it is dead and gone.

Exercise:

Here's an excellent exercise, based on the teaching in The Law of Attraction and some other teachings we have both shared over the years:

- Make a list of the things you want to forgive.
- Write it down.
- Read it out loud.
- Observe your body's reaction when you write and read:

"I forgive _____ for _____. I release all feeling related to this issue and ask that I be healed of all hurt that results from this incident."

- You may notice that when you read this, you get a little twinge of anger or hurt or jealousy. This is a truth indicator, a message that you are doing deep work on an issue you need to address now.

- Do this every day, without fail, until the anger and bitterness have no more hold on you.

- When the issue jumps up again, start the exercise over again with patience and love for yourself.

DR. BEN SAYS: I have a forgiveness issue I've worked on for nearly 20 years now. I lent a guy $20,000 all the way back in 1988. A week later, he filed for bankruptcy. He was planning it and he took my money knowing he would never have to pay it back. I still get a little twitch when I think about it. That means I need to keep working on forgiving him again and again until it's really gone forever.

Self-forgiveness

Self-forgiveness is very tied up in that sense of unworthiness. For most of us, it's harder to find self-forgiveness than to forgive someone else. It's so hard to forgive ourselves for not being what we might have been, for things we might have done or things we did that we wish we had not done.

All of this negative self-talk makes more imprints on our cellular memories and causes more disruption in mental, emotional and physical well-being.

Healing Codes™ to change cellular memories

There is a simple method from *The Healing Codes*™ that will help you dissolve those cellular memories completely.

Dr. Ben and his partner, Dr. Alex Loyd, have graciously agreed to provide us with extensive material from*The Healing Codes*™ and have created a special healing code for breast health.

A little background and explanation first:

The Healing Codes™ were given to Dr. Loyd as an answer to 12 years of fervent prayer for healing for his wife's lifelong and debilitating depression. They are a set of very specifically designed hand positions based on the laws of quantum physics that bring about healing in a new way.

They address those old lies and help re-establish healthy communication between cells by eliminating the lies to forge a sense of self-worth, to forgive others and ourselves, to stop doing harm to ourselves and others, to drop unhealthy belief systems, to love, find joy, peace, patience, kindness, goodness, trust, humility and self-control.

The Healing Codes™ activate a hidden fuse box in the physical body. Think of it this way: Stress breaks the circuit; when the Codes slip the correct switches back on, healing takes place on all levels. It does this by removing the stress from the body, thus allowing the neuroimmune system to take over its job of healing whatever is wrong in the body.

In short, *The Healing Codes*™ work on a physical mechanism built into the body that consistently and predictably removes stress from the body. This is a key point to remember: God designed our bodies to be able to maintain optimal health!

Specially designed Healing Code™ for breast health

Here is a breast health *Healing Code*™ designed specifically for readers of this book to re-establish some of the broken circuits that can negatively impact breast wellness.

The technique is simple:

- The Codes are done by aiming all five fingertips of each hand at the appropriate healing center two or three inches away from the skin. This is much more effective than actually putting your fingertips on the skin because it creates an energy field over the entrance to the healing center.

- It helps to think of your fingertips as tiny flashlights that are shining light on the target area.

- If your arms get tired, you can rest them on a pillow or prop your elbows on a table or on a desk.

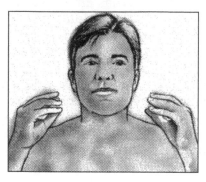 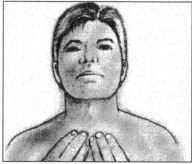

HEALING CODE™ FOR
BREAST HEALTH

Start with a basic prayer for healing. You can devise your own or use this one:

I pray/request that all known and unknown images, beliefs and cellular memories and all resulting physical issues related to my breast health be found, opened and healed by filling me with the love, life and light of God. I also ask that the effectiveness of this healing be increased by one hundred times or more.

1. Aim your fingers at the back corner of your jawbone, a little below the earlobe and then move your fingertips two to three inches out from your body. Hold for 30 seconds.

2. Resting your arms on your chest, aim your fingertips at the healing center at the base of your throat right on the Adam's apple. Hold for 30 seconds.

3. Keep switching between these two positions every 30 seconds until you've been directing the energy for five minutes.

4. Repeat this sequence at least twice a day.

Stress busters

Here's a simple list of ways to de-stress your life:

1. *Recognize what stress feels like.* If you don't recognize that butterflies in the stomach, irritable, talking too much, edgy feeling, work on it. A good stress indicator: shrug your shoulders up to your ears and then drop them back down. You'll probably find you have been carrying your shoulders high and hunched because you are stressed.

2. *Turn off the TV.* Better yet, get it out of the house entirely. The violence, noise and negative messages from television are probably the greatest stressors in our lives and present the most negative influence on our children.

3. *Take a walk.* Any form of exercise is scientifically proven to reduce stress.

4. *Take a deep breath.* Breathing and mental state are intimately linked. If you are stressed, your breathing is undoubtedly quick and shallow. Slow down. Take a few deep long breaths. You'll find your racing mind and stress response will be shifted in seconds.

5. *Do nothing.* Most of us are always doing something. Take a little time every day to do nothing at all.

6. *Find silence.* Pray or meditate. Do whatever it takes to get in touch with your inner stillness. Through the stillness come many answers.

7. *Find some peace and quiet.* This is different from prayer or meditation. It might be a quiet walk in the woods, a bubble bath or some time alone with a good book and a cup of tea.

8. *Nurture.* We know women tend to over nurture, but when your stress threatens to overwhelm you, doing something for someone else can act as a safety valve.

9. *Be nurtured.* Since women are usually the nurturers, it's hard to let go and let someone do something for you. Don't refuse any offer of help. Consider it a gift that would be impolite to refuse.

10. *Set boundaries.* We've mentioned this one before. Learn to say "no" politely and firmly.

11. *Hire a cleaning person.* This one is Kathleen's favorite: She knows from vast experience how stressful it is when the house is a wreck and she's on a book deadline. Give yourself a break at least once a month, more often if you can afford it, and let someone else clean the house.

LAURA'S STORY

Life was all about breasts from the time Laura was six years old and her mother was diagnosed with breast cancer. Through a childhood of care giving until her mother's eventual death when she was 11, through her terror of contracting breast cancer herself; through a marriage in which all of her worth was focused on having beautiful breasts; through breast reduction, removal of a large fibroadenoma tumor and two subsequent implant surgeries with frightening complications — breasts, and her fear that something would go wrong, were the focus of Laura's life.

"I was so terrified of getting breast cancer like my mother did that somewhere in my subconscious mind, I decided I was going to get it," she remembers. "So on my 42nd birthday, the same age when my mother was diagnosed, I got a phone call from my doctor saying that my thermogram showed I was at high risk and on the left side exactly where my mother's cancer was."

Her fears were further fuelled by a really dire family history that gave her a very high risk factor. Not only did Laura's mother die of breast cancer, a couple of her mother's sisters and two cousins also had the disease.

Laura's journey was a lonely one. The little girl cared for her dying mother in every way. She helped bathe her, shave her legs, paint her nails and wax extraneous hair, even while her mother raged about her mastectomy and complained how ugly she looked, grieving over her flat chest and ugly scars.

Since breasts were such a focus in a negative way, it's probably not a surprise that Laura reached thelarche at an early age and had large breasts at age 13.

By the time she was 16, she was so self-conscious about her large breasts that she begged her new stepmother to endorse the idea of breast reduction. Her stepmother strongly disagreed with the idea, as did her doctors.

But that didn't stop the intrepid Laura. Married at 18 to a man who told her he loved her only because of her large breasts, by 21, Laura secretly had breast reduction surgery against her husband's will. Laura went through that surgery alone, without even the support of a sympathetic friend, while her husband went away for the weekend. She was so fearful of her husband's rejection that she began to pad her bras so her smaller breasts would not be noticeable.

"My husband freaked about my breasts. He called them 'two mosquito bites,' even though I was still at least an average D cup," she recalls. "He told me I was lucky he loved me because no one else will ever love me because of the scars."

Before long, Laura was pregnant and her breasts swelled again.

Then came the inevitable day when her emotionally and verbally abusive alcoholic husband told her she bored him.

"I had kids, no schooling, and I thought 'Oh, my gosh, if I make myself more beautiful, he'll love me again," Laura remembers.

Laura became a "workout queen" obsessing about her gym time, getting her BMI (body mass index) into the lower 20s. Of course, as Laura lost weight and built muscle mass, her breasts got a little smaller and her husband was angry with her. At this time she was diagnosed with a fibroadenoma tumor in the left breast and had to have it out. Now her breasts were uneven.

So Laura underwent a third surgery, this one to make her breasts symmetrical and even. Where once she thought her breasts were too large, she had made a 180-degree turn and decided they were not perfect in her husband's eyes so she scheduled implant surgery.

"I realize now that all of my feelings of self-worth were tied up in my breasts. I was obsessing about them constantly," Laura says.

"A week after the implant surgery, I got an infection and the horror of everything my mother went through and the fear of losing my breast just like my mother put me in a state of absolute panic," she continues. "I was alone in the hospital for 3 1/2 weeks getting mega antibiotic therapy trying to save the implant. No one was allowed to know. My husband told people I had a mental breakdown and no one could see me. I spent endless nights crying and feeling very alone. My self-esteem was as low as it could get."

She was finally released from the hospital, still in immense pain, but unable to persuade any of her doctors that something was still not right.

Eventually her husband's prophecy came true and she did suffer an emotional breakdown. She was placed in a psychiatric ward for several days so she could "calm down." Everyone told her that the pain was in her head.

But nothing was wrong with Laura's mind that proper medical treatment wouldn't solve.

After months of suffering, she told her best friend about the pain she was still experiencing, and her friend encouraged her to visit another doctor who immediately diagnosed an infection behind the chest wall, caused by one of the implants. The implant had to come out.

"My breast had swollen to the size of a cantaloupe, I had to have the implant out," Laura says. "I drove myself again to the hospital alone and scared, with no support from my husband."

The infection caused her to lose so much breast tissue that her breast became flattened and shapeless.

Undaunted, Laura went back for more surgery just six months later. She got another infection, but with quick medical intervention and another surgery, the implants and her breast were saved.

In the interim, Laura had some realizations about the destructive nature of her marriage and had extricated herself from it.

She spent several years getting herself on her feet, regaining her self-esteem, getting training to become a massage therapist and energy worker and mending her relationship with her children. All of these efforts were fruitful, but Laura's terror of losing her breasts continued to consume her.

Her breakthrough came about a year after the high risk thermogram results came in.

"A friend dragged me off to a *Healing Codes*™: seminar," she laughs. "I didn't want to go. My back was hurting like crazy and I was really cranky throughout the whole first day.

The second day she made a connection with Dr. Ben who noticed her back pain and offered some solace.

Laura gives credit to Dr. Ben and *The Healing Codes*™: "From then on, Dr. Ben became my coach. He's worked me through the anger, unforgiveness and fear. I've worked my way through *The Healing Codes*™: and I'm clear now. My fear of cancer is gone."

By working *The Healing Codes*™: and releasing those cellular memories of fear and anger and unworthiness, Laura can proudly point to a physical milestone: Her most recent thermogram showed her at medium risk for breast cancer, a far sight better than her high risk result just two years ago.

DR. BEN SAYS: Laura is one of the most remarkable women I have ever met. The amount of work she has done, the courage and the will she has presented to overcome the issues of her life are truly an inspiration.

Chapter 8 BREAST CANCER: WHO'S AT HIGHEST RISK? HOW CAN YOU REDUCE YOUR RISK?

Women worry about breast cancer. There is such an innate fear of this disease that fear itself increases the risk of developing the disease.

Yes, women are at risk for breast cancer. Yes, the risk increases with age. Yes, breast cancer is the number one cancer killer of white and African-American women. And yes, 99 percent of those who contract breast cancer are women.

More than 212,000 women in the United States were diagnosed with breast cancer in 2006 and about 40,000 died of the disease.

And the numbers are growing rapidly. In 1960, an average woman's lifetime chance of getting breast cancer was one in 20; today, it is one in eight. We'll go more deeply into the reasons in Chapter 9, but let us suggest one more time that the increasing toxic load on our bodies, especially the harmful environmental estrogens or xenoestrogens, are almost certainly an underlying factor in this frightening increase in the number of cases of breast cancer.

And while the incidence of breast cancer is increasing, it's important to put these numbers in perspective. More than 500,000 women die of heart disease every year. This is in excess of 12 times the number of deaths caused by breast cancer and more than double the number of women who die of all types of cancer. That doesn't mean you shouldn't pay attention to breast health. Of course you should. That's why we have written this book. Yet women seem to have less

BREAST CANCER RISK SURVEY

1. How old are you?
   A. 15-35
   B. 36-50
   C. 50-65
   D. 65 or over

2. Have you ever been tested for the BRCA1 and BRCA2 genes?
   A. Yes
   B. No

3. If you've been tested, did the results show you were positive for either of these genes?
   A. Yes
   B. No

4. Do you have a mother, sister or daughter who has had breast cancer?
   A. Yes
   B. No

5. Do you smoke?
   A. Yes
   B. No

6. How tall are you?
   A. Under 5'2"
   B. 5'3" to 5'6"
   C. 5'7" or more

7. Are you overweight?
   A. Yes
   B. No

8. If you are overweight, how many pounds are you above your ideal weight?
   A. 5-15
   B. 16-25
   C. 26-50
   D. 50 or more

9. Do you drink alcoholic beverages?
   A. Yes
   B. No

10. If yes, how many drinks do you have on the average day?
    A. 0-1
    B. 2-3
    C. 4 or more

11. What is the average number of serving of fruits and vegetables you eat per day (not including potatoes)?
    A. 0-2
    B. 2-4
    C. 5-7
    D. 8 or more

12. How old were you when you had your first menstrual period?
    A. 8-9
    B. 10-11
    C. 12-14
    D. 15 or over

13. What is your race?
    A. Caucasian
    B. African American
    C. Hispanic
    D. Asian-Pacific Islander
    E. Other

14. Are you of Ashkenazi-Jewish descent?
    A. Yes
    B. No

15. How many times have you been pregnant?
    A. 0
    B. 1-2
    C. 3 or more

16. Have you ever had an abortion?
    A. Yes
    B. No

17. How many live births have you had?
    D. 0
    E. 1-2
    F. 3 or more

18. Did you breast feed your children?
    a. Yes
    b. No

19. If yes, what was the total number of months you breast fed your children?
    a. 1-3 months
    b. 4-6 months
    c. 6-12 months
    d. 13 months or more

20. Have you taken birth control pills or used the birth control patch?
    a. Yes
    b. No

21. If yes, how long was your total use of the pill or patch?
    a. 1 year or less
    b. 1-2 years
    c. 2-4 years
    d. 4 years or more

22. What is your menopausal state?
    a. I'm not menopausal
    b. Perimenopausal (starting into menopausal changes)
    c. Post menopausal

23. If you are perimenopausal or menopausal, at what age did you become fully menopausal (no periods for 12 months)?
    a. 40 or under
    b. 41-50
    c. 50 or older

24. Have you ever taken hormone replacement therapy?
    a. Yes
    b. No

25. If yes, what type did you take?
    a. Synthetic
    b. Conjugated equine estrogens (i.e. Premarin™ or PremPro™)
    c. Synthetic progesterone (Provera™)

    d. edroxyprogesterone acetate (MPA)
    e. Estratab™, Menest™
    f. Ogen™, Ortho-est™
    g. Bioidentical hormones

26. Have you had a hysterectomy?
    a. Yes
    b. No

27. Have you ever had a breast biopsy?
    a. Yes
    b. No

28. Have you ever been diagnosed with any type of cancer?
    a. Yes
    b. No

29. Have you ever had radiation therapy?
    a. Yes
    b. No

30. Have you had extensive chest X-rays or other types of radiation in the chest area, especially when you were young?
    a. Yes
    b. No

31. Have you ever been diagnosed with breast hyperplasia?
    a. Yes
    b. No

32. Have you ever taken an extensive course of antibiotics?
    a. Yes
    b. No

33. Did you take antibiotics for a total of more than 100 days before the age of 18?
    a. Yes
    b. No

34. Do you wear a bra more than 12 hours a day?
    a. Yes
    b. No

fear of heart disease than they have of breast cancer, perhaps because women have less information on heart disease. Stay tuned for a coming book in this series on women and heart health.

Having a risk factor for breast cancer, or even several, does not mean that you will get the disease. The vast majority of women who have one or more breast cancer risk factor never develop the disease. On the other hand, many women with breast cancer have no apparent risk factors (other than being a woman and growing older). Even when a woman with breast cancer has a risk factor, there is no way to prove that it actually caused her cancer.

There are several types of risk factors. Some you cannot control, such as your sex, age and race. And some, like smoking, drinking, diet and stress, you can control.

Please see the brief risk assessment questionnaire on page 92 and then we will examine in detail the risk factors for breast cancer and their relative seriousness.

How important are the risk factors?

Before we launch into a detailed description of risk factors, we want to put the whole picture in perspective.

The majority of women with breast cancer don't have any risk factors.

Risk factors are important, and if you have them, do whatever you can to diminish them.

Obsessing with fear about getting breast cancer sends an unhealthy message to the cells where it becomes implanted in your cellular memory.

This chapter and the ones that follow are meant to educate you, not to instill fear in you. Knowledge is power. When you are armed with knowledge, you can make healthy choices.

The risks and what they mean

We're not going to give you a specific score for your risks. Instead, please read this section carefully and figure for yourself whether you are at high or low risk and then act accordingly.

The scientific community will tell you that the greatest risk for breast cancer is a woman's lifetime exposure to estrogen. In general, we agree with that.

However, it's very important here to point out that the cellular memories, the stressors in your life, conscious or unconscious, are disrupting communications between cells and increasing the risk of all types of diseases.

So, what does "lifetime exposure to estrogen" mean?

It means the amount of estrogen to which you are exposed in your lifetime from menarche to menopause, pregnancies and miscarriages or abortions, birth control pills, breast feeding and hormone replacement therapy.

It's more difficult to assess your exposure to xenoestrogens and the risks they pose. While we haven't included it in the questionnaire, the amount of red meat and dairy products you eat can be considered a risk factor, although we think the risk has more to do with the hormones that are given to beef and dairy cattle and the plastic and Styrofoam packaging in which it is sold than anything else. It is possible you can somewhat neutralize that risk by eating more antioxidant-rich fruits and vegetables.

Being female: While men can develop breast cancer, 99 percent of those with breast cancer are women. This is probably because men have comparatively little breast tissue and while men do have estrogen in their bodies, the amounts are comparatively small.

Age: As you age, your risk of breast cancer increases. If you're under 40, the risk is relatively small and it is the highest in those 70 years old and older. From birth to age 39, the risk is 1 in 231 or 0.5 percent. From the ages of 40 to 59, the risk is 1 in 25 or 4 percent. From age 60 to 79, the chance is 1 in 15 or nearly 7 percent. If you live to the age of 90, your chance of getting breast cancer over an entire lifetime is 1 in 7, with an overall lifetime risk of 14.3 percent.

Family history: If your first degree blood relatives (mother, sister or daughter) have breast cancer, your chances of developing the disease are doubled. If more than one first degree relative has had breast cancer, your chances are increased five-fold. The risk increases if your relative's cancer was diagnosed before she was 50 years old.

In the genes: Some women with a strong family history of the disease have inherited a genetic abnormality that increases their risk for breast cancer. So far, abnormalities that have been found to have a definite link to an increased risk for breast cancer are in the BRCA1 and BRCA2 genes. Studies have shown that for such women, breast cancer risk could be as high as 80 to 90 percent by the age of 70. Some women have opted to take preventive measures, including mastectomy, double mastectomy, ovary removal, and Tamoxifen™ therapy. These are all very serious measures that can significantly change a woman's life.

Height: Taller women have a higher risk of breast cancer, although scientists don't know exactly why. One simple reason may be that the taller you are, the more cells you have in your body, increasing the number of cells that could become cancerous. It may also be that taller people grow faster as children and that type of fast growth is linked to changes in the DNA of the cells, which may become cancerous.

Weight: Maintaining a healthy weight helps protect you from breast cancer, especially if you are postmenopausal. Losing weight lowers the amount of estrogen in a woman's body and reduces that lifetime exposure to estrogen we were talking about earlier. While most estrogen comes from the ovaries during a woman's reproductive life, estrogen after menopause is released by fat cells, so the fewer fat cells you have, the lower your estrogen load and the less your risk of breast cancer. The risk is especially great for women who gain weight as adults and especially applies to weight gain after menopause. Carrying excess weight in the abdomen, rather than in the thighs or buttocks is an additional risk factor.

Diet: This probably won't come as much of a surprise. The more vegetables you eat, the lower your risk of virtually every type of cancer and breast cancer is on that list. Scientists theorize that the decreased risk may be due to the antioxidants in fruits and vegetables, especially those rich in vitamin A.

Alcohol: There is a very fine line on the health benefits and health risks of alcohol consumption and breast cancer. Several studies show that women who drink one drink a day have a lower risk of breast cancer (and heart disease and diabetes) than women who do not drink at all or women who drink more than one drink a day. Red wine rich in antioxidants is especially beneficial. Just going over that fine line to two drinks a day can increase your risk.

Smoking: Researchers think that higher estrogen levels combined with cancer-causing agents in tobacco spark the development of breast tumors. Smoking definitely increases the risk of breast cancer.

Age at menarche: The earlier a girl has her first menstrual period, the greater her risk of breast cancer, since her lifetime estrogen exposure is greater. Girls today are reaching menarche at a younger age than their grandmothers and their mothers, so they are at higher risk.

Various studies linking birth control pills and the risk of breast cancer have produced conflicting results. One study of more than 100,000 women suggests that the increased breast cancer risk associated with birth control pills is highest among women over age 45 who were still using the pill. This group of women was nearly one-and-a-half times as likely to get breast cancer as women who had never used the pill, probably because of the long-term exposure to estrogen.

Abortion: This is not in any way meant to be a value judgment for what is an extremely difficult decision for any woman. It is a simple medical assessment of the risks further down the road for women who have had an abortion. When a pregnancy is abruptly terminated, a woman's hormones quite literally fall off the cliff. In the early stages of pregnancy, cells are dividing extremely rapidly as the fetus grows. The woman's entire physiological structure is geared to supporting that fast growth and new life. The glandular system in the breast is extra sensitive at this time because it is preparing to breast feed a child. So when there is no longer a reason to support that rapid cell division for a developing fetus, the body is left in an exceptionally estrogen sensitive state and it can become confused and bring about that cell division elsewhere, in a malignant tumor. Women who have abortions are also vulnerable because of the emotional stress that usually accompanies the decision to terminate a pregnancy.

Age at birth of first child: The younger a woman is when she has her first child, the lower her risk of developing breast cancer during her lifetime. A woman who has her first child after the age of 30 has approximately twice the risk of developing breast cancer as a woman who gave birth before her 21st birthday, and about the same risk as a woman who has never given birth. In addition, the more children a woman has, the lower her risk of breast cancer. While we know this statistically, scientists aren't sure why this is the case, but the hormones associated with pregnancy probably play a role.

Number of pregnancies: Women who have more than one child have a lower risk of developing breast cancer.

Breast biopsies: Women who have had breast biopsies have an increased risk of breast cancer, especially if the biopsy showed a change in breast tissue, known as atypical hyperplasia. These women are at increased risk because of whatever prompted the biopsies, not because of the biopsies themselves.

Previous breast cancer diagnosis: The risk of cancer returning or appearing in the other breast is substantial for women who have been diagnosed with cancer. There are many factors, but the risk is generally considered to diminish the longer a woman remains cancer-free.

Menopausal status: Women who are not fully menopausal until after the age of 55 are at a higher risk. We've already gone into synthetic hormone replacement in greater detail, but this type of hormone replacement clearly increases a woman's risk of breast cancer during the menopausal years.

Race: White women have greater risk of developing breast cancer than African-American women (although black women diagnosed with breast cancer are more likely to die of the disease because they are usually at a more advanced stage when they are diagnosed.) Women of Ashkenazi Jewish descent have a higher risk of breast cancer. Scientists are uncertain why this is the case.

Income: Women of all races with incomes below the poverty level are more often diagnosed with late-stage breast cancer and more likely to die of the disease than are women with higher incomes. This is because low-income women often don't receive the routine medical care that would allow breast cancer to be discovered earlier.

Breast density: On X-rays, dense breast tissue looks solid and white, so it can mask tumors. Increasingly, breast density is often recognized as a breast cancer risk factor in and of itself. The abundant glandular tissue in dense breasts means there are many more cells with the potential to become cancerous. Your age and menopausal status affect your breast density. Younger women tend to have denser breasts.

Radiation exposure: If you received radiation treatments to your chest as a child or as a young adult, or you had a number of chest or spinal x-rays, your risk of developing breast cancer later in life is increased.

Antibiotics: Research shows that women who took antibiotics for more than 500 days or who had more than 25 prescriptions in the course of a 17-year period more than doubled their risk of breast cancer compared with women who had not taken large amounts of antibiotics.

Bras: Women who wear a bra more than 12 hours a day increase their risk by 20 times! This was discussed at length in Chapter 3. It is a risk factor you can easily control and we highly recommend ditching your bra, if you can, or wearing one as few hours of the day as possible.

Chapter 9 I'VE FOUND A LUMP. NOW WHAT?

So, you're doing your monthly breast self-exam (BSE) right on schedule and—wait! Your heart skips a beat. There's something that wasn't there last month. You're sure. That hard little lump deep in the top of your left breast is new.

Heart pounding a little more wildly, you fight down a feeling of panic. Maybe you drink a glass of wine and think about what you should do.

Your first action was absolutely correct. A glass of wine, a little reflection and a calm response are essential when you find yourself in this situation.

You might want to ask your partner to check the suspect place and get an amateur "second opinion."

Sleep on it, one night only. Don't panic, but don't procrastinate.

In all of his years of clinical practice, Dr. Ben has treated thousands of women, many of them who have discovered suspicious lumps in their breasts. He always respects their knowledge of their bodies and their sense that there is something "different." Your doctor should, too.

Look for a team player

Your next step is to find a physician who is willing to play on your team. Be sure the doctor understands it is your team and your breast and your life that is at stake. You are in control!

Kathleen says she looks at the process of finding the right doctor much like hiring someone to fix her computer: You are hiring someone with some very specialized knowledge to do a job for you. You are quite literally hiring someone to work for you. You are paying your doctor to give you the best possible medical advice. But it is your body, it is your life and you are in charge. Anything less is simply not acceptable.

The days of doctors playing God are long gone. With the advent of the Internet, patients have access to loads of information (granted, some of it is inaccurate) and have the potential and the responsibility to inform themselves.

Run away as fast as you can from a doctor who pats you on the head and says, "Don't worry, honey, I'll take care of everything."

You have a right to have your condition and your options explained to you in simple-to-understand English. You have a right to know the possible consequences of certain decisions you might make. But you and you alone will make the final decision on how you will approach this based on the information you have hired your doctor to give you.

You don't have a right to expect your doctor to perform miracles or to swear on a stack of Bibles you'll get cured. That's not possible and it's not fair.

You can expect your doctor to take your side, to treat you as an individual and not as a "case" or a diagnosis, if it comes to that. You have a right to expect your doctor to research your options carefully and to seek the opinions of colleagues who are experts in your particular medical problem. You also have the right to request a referral to an oncologist (a cancer specialist), if you wish.

Once you have firmly established that relationship with your doctor, you'll probably be asked to undergo some more testing.

What's next?

The first thing any doctor will want to do when you say you have found a lump is to examine it personally. This exam will be quite similar to your monthly BSE. It is nearly the same as the routine clinical examination that is done every time you visit your gynecologist/family physician for an annual checkup.

Ultrasound

The next step probably should be to get an ultrasound. An ultrasound will determine if the lump you have found is a fluid-filled cyst or if it is a hard mass.

How the ultrasound works: It shows the outlines of the lump (unless it is very deep, in which case, it would be unlikely that you would have been able to feel it). Imagine there is a small water balloon inside there. When pressure is applied to the water balloon, it will dent in and then go back to its original position when the pressure is released. If this is what happens, you can breathe a sigh of relief. You have a fluid-filled cyst. These are almost always non-cancerous.

If the lump appears to be a cyst, and if you are so inclined, you can have a needle aspiration. This is a simple procedure that usually takes place in the doctor's office. The breast is numbed and a needle guided into the cyst and the fluid drawn out. The cyst will collapse like an old balloon and the outer walls will eventually be re-absorbed by your body.

Just to be entirely sure you won't have further problems, the fluid drawn from the cyst will be analyzed for cancer cells.

With suspected cysts, many doctors will recommend waiting a month or two to see if the lump disappears on its own, which is frequently the case. Checking the lump during a different part of your menstrual cycle may also be helpful.

If the ultrasound shows a solid mass, you and your doctor will need to gather more information.

Try for an MRI

Finding a solid mass is definitely a cause for concern. We are not in any way suggesting that you ignore it or "wait and see."

You must be proactive immediately.

Your first move should be to get an MRI. This scan uses radio frequency signals to give doctors a good look at the inside of your body. There is no radiation unlike in a CT scan, which uses a specialized type of X-ray. MRIs are not infallible, but they can provide more information about the size and location of a mass. The National Cancer Institute says MRIs cannot always distinguish between a malignant tumor and a benign one.

The next step will probably be a diagnostic mammogram. This may sound contradictory, but we agree that this is the time for a mammogram. Mammograms can be a valuable diagnostic tool. Yes, they do deliver a whopping amount of radiation, but this is the time to do whatever you need to do to get the answers you need.

Just say "No!" to a biopsy

This is where conventional medicine and Dr. Ben part ways, big time.

Most conventional doctors will want you to undergo a needle biopsy as a next step in the diagnostic process. Dr. Ben urges you in the most emphatic terms, "Say NO!"

A biopsy is a way of taking a sample of tens of thousands of cells from the tumor by inserting a needle into the mass.

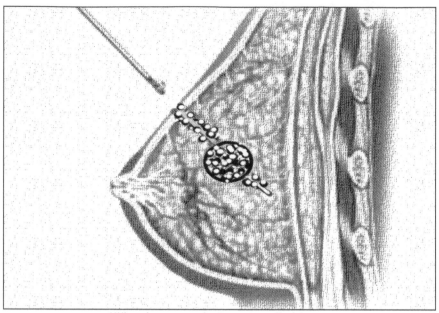

What happens during a needle biopsy

The act of inserting that needle into the mass penetrates the outer edges of the mass and can "seed" cells out the other side of the mass or bring them with the needle as it is withdrawn. Potentially leaving them in healthy tissue.

The only "good" type of biopsy

If you feel you must have a biopsy and you are prepared to go into surgery knowing that your breast will be removed if a cancer diagnosis comes back from the lab while you are on the operating table, excisional biopsy (also known as lumpectomy) is the option you should choose. It's also sometimes called a whole sample biopsy because the whole lump is removed without touching it.

This is a surgical procedure, performed in a hospital under anesthesia, in which an incision is made in the breast and the entire mass is removed and sent to the lab while you are still asleep. If the lab report comes back that the mass is malignant, the breast is immediately removed. This is the only method to definitively diagnose breast cancer without the procedure causing more harm than good.

If you are mentally and emotionally prepared for the possibility that you could wake up from surgery and learn your breast has been removed, an excisional biopsy can give you a great deal of peace of mind.

After an excisional biopsy, assuming the results are in your favor, you'll have a small scar and likely there will be a dimple in your breast. The size of the dimple depends on the size of the mass that was removed and the dimple often becomes nearly indistinguishable in large-breasted women.

If you have had a mastectomy, read the information about mastectomy and breast reconstructive surgery in Chapter 11.

ELIZABETH EDWARDS' STORY

The story of Elizabeth Edwards, wife of former senator and presidential candidate John Edwards and an intelligent and dynamic person in her own right, is an excellent case in point. In 2004, the day before the election in which her husband was a vice-presidential candidate, Elizabeth found a large lump in her breast.

Immediately after the votes were counted, she had a lumpectomy and several rounds of chemotherapy and radiation – the standard treatment.

Elizabeth and her family believed she was cancer free, a sad but common delusion. I've seen so many cancer patients clutch at that hope that "they got it all."

I'm sure her doctors told Elizabeth she was tumor free, not cancer free. No doctor can guarantee that someone is cancer free and no doctor should.

If you're treading this treacherous pathway, you need to understand something very important here about doctor-talk: Elizabeth Edwards was never "in remission." That was smoke and mirrors. She simply did not have a cell mass big enough for doctors to detect.

In fact, I think most of us have cancer cells in our bodies most of the time. Whether they ever develop into something to concern us depends on many things, including our cellular memories and our ability to combat the abnormal cell growth.

With Elizabeth Edwards' case, almost inevitably cells migrated to her bones and lungs, common sites for breast cancer metastasis, before her breast cancer was ever discovered.

As I write this, two and one-half years after the diagnosis, Elizabeth's cancer has returned. A small mass has been found on her rib and several tiny spots on her lungs. It is terribly sad, but one good thing is that these are inoperable, so doctors will be able to use these spots as

---

> mirrors to see if their prescribed treatment is working.
>
> I pray for Elizabeth and all breast cancer survivors to have long, healthy lives. My heart goes out to her husband and her children. Certainly this wonderful woman's life span will be considerably shorter than all of them would have hoped.

Creating a mirror

If a biopsy suggests a mass is malignant, standard medical practice calls for the mass to be surgically removed in a procedure called either a lumpectomy (removing the lump) or mastectomy (removing the entire breast and nearby lymph glands and nodes).

This may seem counter-intuitive, however, Dr. Ben thinks this is an incorrect approach. He is strongly in favor of leaving the mass in place so it can act as a mirror for other cells that might have migrated to other parts of the body.

The problem with removing the lump is that you have removed your means of determining what is happening with those other microscopic cells that may take 5 to 10 years to become visible to any means available to standard medicine like CT scans, MRIs, PET scans, and bone scans.

A tumor is defined as a solid mass of cells. The smallest sized tumors detectable by mammograms, MRIs and PET scans are one centimeter or about 3/8 of an inch.

If you remove a cancerous lump, you have removed the mirror that can show you how well your treatment is working in the breast and in all other parts of your body where there may be tiny clusters of cells beginning to grow that may not be detectable for years to come.

We'll go into this further in Chapter 11, but let it suffice for now to say that diligent monitoring of the size of the lump will indicate to you whether traditional therapies like chemotherapy and radiation are working and the effectiveness of herbal, homeopathic or other complementary therapies if you are going that route.

If you take out this "mirror," you don't have a clue whether your treatment is working until years later and you've done four or five PET scans and suddenly a tumor mass grows to the size where these machines can see it. A one-centimeter tumor has about a billion cells in it. You can see why you don't want to wait for that to be detectable!

Check your thermogram

Thermograms are not diagnostic tools for breast cancer, but they are most definitely a source of important information. If you've had baseline thermograms, you have been alerted to an abnormal growth that indicates an increased blood flow to cells that might be cancerous. Thermograms offer the best option to take preventive measures long before a tumor visible to medical science ever develops.

As we told you in Chapter 5, by detecting the blood supply in the breast and the "off the grid" nature of blood supply to cancerous growth, thermograms can tell what might happen years down the road, long before mammograms, MRIs and ultrasounds can pick it up.

If you haven't had baseline thermograms and you have a suspicious mass, a thermogram can tell you and your doctor exactly where you are today. It can also chart any growth or shrinkage of the blood vessel supply to the mass when it's repeated in three or six months or a year. A thermogram is an important non-invasive and radiation-free component to any plan to use the mass in a breast as a mirror to determine the effectiveness of treatment.

A thermogram is an early warning system to tell you that you may be headed for trouble. This gives you ample opportunity to change your diet and your lifestyle, and, most importantly, to change the way you are thinking and not fall into fear and panic that will imbed new and powerful cellular memories that will further compromise your immune system and impair your body's ability to fight off the cancerous invader.

Blood tests

It would be wonderful if we could say that a simple blood test will absolutely give you a "Yes" or "No" answer, but it's not that easy, since there are so many different types of cancer cells and they act in so many different ways.

However, there are a number of blood tests that might be helpful in reaching a diagnosis. It is definitely worthwhile for you and your doctor to examine the possibilities.

As body cells die at the end of their natural life cycle, their contents dissolve and they are scavenged by the lymphatic system and carried through the blood. Tumor markers are looking for identifiable little pieces of those cells in the blood.

Probably the best blood test and the most accurate one for people in early stages of breast cancer is the *AMAS* (Anti-Malignan Antibody in Serum) test. This is a relatively new test that measures specific blood antibodies (proteins in the blood that help the body fight disease) called malignans. Malignan antibody levels are higher in people with early stage breast cancer, so this blood test can be helpful in early detection. AMAS can also be helpful in determining the return of cancer once treatment is complete. Research showed that in control groups of women with known breast cancer, the test was 96 percent accurate.

You've probably heard of the *CA-125* test that measures for blood antigens (molecules that trigger immune responses) for hormonally-related cancers, like breast cancer. It is a good test, but it is not very effective at all in the early stages of breast cancer. CA-125 is most reliable in very advanced cancers. Other markers called CA 15-3 and CEA (Carcinoembryonic antigen) are also used to measure advanced breast cancer, but are not very helpful in early stages of the disease.

Blood tests measuring mammoglobulin, a protein found in malignant breast tumors, is helpful in determining if cancer has spread to other parts of the body with nearly 80 percent accuracy.

The *HER2* gene test detects the overgrowth of a certain type of protein and/or the presence of gene-based hormone overproduction that can contribute to the growth of cancer cells and the spread of these cells to other parts of the body.

Another gene, the *P53*, stops cells with DNA damage from multiplying until the DNA is repaired or the cell dies. If the P53 gene is damaged or malfunctioning, that control is lost and cancerous cells can multiply, so testing for P53 damage may provide helpful information.

S Phase is another gene test that can determine if the substances that govern exact reproduction of cells have become damaged, allowing tumors to grow.

It may not be cancer at all

It's important to remember that 90 percent of breast lumps are not cancerous. Keep your perspective and realize that, even if something is wrong, it is very likely that it is not cancer.

Fibrocystic breast disease: One of the most common breast conditions was until recently called fibrocystic breast disease. However, doctors found that this condition, unscientifically called lumpy breasts, is common, harmless and affects 60 percent of all women. It is now officially called fibrocystic breast condition. It is most pronounced between the ages of 30 and 50, and the problem usually diminishes after menopause. Women with fibrocystic breasts complain that their breasts become painful and the lumpiness is more pronounced at certain times of their menstrual cycles as hormones ebb and flow. Some researchers argue that women with fibrocystic breasts are more susceptible to breast cancer, but the research is far from conclusive on that issue. It's important to pay attention if you have fibrocystic breasts simply because the normal lumpiness may cause a woman to overlook a suspicious lump. While the cause of fibrocystic breasts is unknown, the symptoms may diminish if you decrease your intake of caffeine, nicotine and theophylline, a compound found in tea. Supplementation with SSKI, a saturated solution of potassium iodide is also helpful. Two drops in a glass of water a day should do it. A word of caution; this is definitely a situation where more is not better. Too much potassium iodide can affect your thyroid. You should be able to get SSKI from your local pharmacist without a prescription.

Cysts: We've already mentioned cysts, but it's worth going a little more deeply into the subject here. These fluid-filled oval shaped sacs are found in about one-third of all women between the ages of 35 and 50. A soft, round, moveable lump, especially if it is tender to the touch, is most likely a cyst. They often enlarge and become painful just before a woman's menstrual period because of the hormonal changes. Cysts are usually diagnosed by ultrasound and they can be safely drained by inserting a needle into the sac and drawing out the fluid. They are almost never cancerous, but any drained fluid should be examined by a laboratory.

Fibroadenoma: These hard, rubbery tumors are smooth and easily moveable, unlike cancerous tumors which are most often bumpy and rooted. They usually occur in younger women under the age of 30. They are small, usually not more than an inch in diameter. They often disappear without treatment. The cause of fibroadenomas is not known, but some experts theorize that there may be an estrogen component since they often become larger in the late phases of the menstrual cycle and they usually disappear after a woman reaches menopause. Fibroadenomas are usually diagnosed by a doctor's clinical examination because of the characteristic smoothness and moveabiity. Sometimes an ultrasound will confirm the diagnosis. Fibroadenomas are not cancerous and rarely become cancerous.

Calcifications: These common calcium deposits appear as white lumps on mammograms, since the radiation cannot pass through them. They are not cancerous in and of themselves, but certain patterns of calcification can indicate the presence of breast cancer. Since we know that cancers deposit calcium, these calcifications get our attention. When they appear as large white dots or dashes, they are usually not a cause for concern and may indicate clogging of a milk duct, the result of an injury, inflammation caused by an infection or even the clogging of an artery.

> **IF YOU ARE DEALING WITH
> AN UNDIAGNOSED LUMP
> IN YOUR BREAST,
> YOU NEED TO EAT AND LIVE
> AS IF YOU HAVE CANCER,
> BUT THINK
> IN YOUR SPIRIT,
> "I AM FREE AND
> I AM HEALTHY."**

Chapter 10 WHAT IS BREAST CANCER? WHERE DOES IT COME FROM? HOW DOES CONVENTIONAL MEDICINE TREAT IT?

All cells in the human body have a natural life span. They are born, hopefully, as exact copies of their parent cells, they perform their functions and they die.

Sometimes that perfect system gets disrupted; something goes wrong and cells literally lose their identities. They lose track of what kind of cell they really are and they forget how to perform their function and die in a normal fashion.

They reproduce too fast, don't do their jobs correctly, if at all, they live far longer than they should, and their offspring aren't exact copies of the parent cells.

Those hyperactive cells tend to clump together, forming tumors.

All cancers are caused by genetic miscues, but only 5 to 10 percent of them are caused by the genes you inherited from your parents and 90 percent are due to the imperfect copying of genes that is the result of aging, lifestyle, diet and, you guessed it: cellular memories that cause a disconnect from the perfect genetic material that could help us live healthy lives, perhaps for over a hundred years.

It's essential to stop these cancerous cells from growing and to change the toxic environment that caused those cells to become cancerous. The cancer would not have been able to grow in a healthy environment.

Malignant tumors in the breast are closely linked to hormones, and particularly to estrogen. That's why women bear 99 percent of the burden of breast cancer, although it does rarely occur in men, since men have estrogen and breast tissue, too.

The process of aging and a woman's lifetime exposure to estrogen are her greatest risks for developing breast cancer.

By the way, estrogen isn't always a bad guy. Estrogen is what allows a woman to form eggs, become pregnant, carry a baby and give birth. It's also an essential component of bone growth, helps with digestive functions, promotes healthy blood clotting, normalizes cholesterol and keeps fluids in balance. Women need it. Without estrogen, the human race would die out in one generation.

Yet too much estrogen throughout a lifetime is a known cancer risk and also increases the risks of heart disease, stroke and Alzheimer's.

Statistics

Every three minutes, an American woman is diagnosed with breast cancer. In 2006, an estimated 212,920 new cases of invasive breast cancer were diagnosed along with 612,980 cases of noninvasive breast cancer. Breast cancer was expected to claim the lives of 40,970 women and men in 2006. Yet about 400,000 women are living today with breast cancer.

Perhaps most disheartening, the rate of breast cancer was one in 20 women in 1960. Today it is one in 8.

EXERCISE TO ACCESS A CELLULAR MEMORY

Take a moment to close your eyes and sit quietly. Now call up a memory of something you haven't thought about in a long time, perhaps your second grade teacher or your best friend when you were ten years old or a family picnic when you were five. That memory will pop up from your memory hard drive. Where did it come from? You might feel the excitement of winning the pin-the-tail-on-the-donkey or the mellow comfort of having a friend. Where was that memory stored? Not just in your brain. It is stored in every cell of your body. That is cellular memory, a term often used in quantum physics, the science of the tiniest particles ever discovered and their tremendous effect on the universe.

Breast cancer causes more deaths among Caucasian and African-American women than any other type of cancer. Jewish women of Ashkenazi descent, which account for about 90 percent of Jewish women in the U.S., are at a higher risk than Caucasian women. Asian-American women have a lower risk, as do Hispanics and Native Americans.

If all this seems like a lot of bad news, consider this: The death rates have declined significantly every year in the 1990s, the most recent years for which statistics are available.

Cancer and the Law of Attraction

All the way back in 1971, President Richard Nixon declared war on cancer. At the time, cancer was the eighth leading cause of death in America.

Now, 37 years later and with hundreds of billions of dollars spent on research, cancer has become the second leading cause of death in America. For one brief terrible moment, cancer was the leading cause of death.

Are we winning this war?

Not really.

Why not?

Dr. Ben has four explanations:

1. *Stress:* We've talked about this in earlier chapters. Modern life has resulted in a huge increase in stress across the board. No one escapes in this fast-paced society. We work longer and harder. Work always beckons through cell phones, blackberries and laptops. Kathleen says this is why she loves to scuba dive, since there are no cell phones at the bottom of the ocean...or is there some new technology that she hasn't heard about yet that will invade even that silent paradise? One week of the New York Times contains more information than a person received in an entire lifetime just 100 years ago. We have almost no "down time" anymore. We are seldom alone. This emotional stress leads to a cascade of physical responses that leaves us vulnerable, with our immune systems unable to bring those rogue cells back in line.

2. *Toxic environment:* The external toxins we take into our bodies have without a doubt increased the cancer rate, especially as we become more vulnerable through high stress levels. From air pollution to the pollution of water supplies to radiation to the ever-present xenoestrogens in meat, dairy products and plastics, we are building

horrifying toxic loads in our bodies and the environment. Frequently, the toxins tip the balance and allow the growth of cancerous cells.

3. *Viral load:* There is a virus in every cancer cell that has contributed to the cell running amok. Most cancer patients Dr. Ben has treated carry viral loads from cytomegalovirus virus, herpes simplex virus (HSV) or human papillomavirus (HPV), all of which are transmitted through body fluids and are therefore preventable. And all of them affect between 80 and 90 percent of the population by age 50. Once we've been exposed, these viruses remain in our bodies forever and cause periodic outbreaks, sometimes aggravated by stress. These and many other viruses become a distraction to lower the body's awareness of cancer cells in the first place and to forget to fight them in the second place. The continuous battle against these viruses exhausts the immune system and opens the door to many diseases, including cancer.

4. *Memory toxicity:* Television and movies are having the most profound effect of all. Those scenes of murder, rape, plunder and pillage are all being stored in our cellular memories. Every movie we see, every rape or murder is stored somewhere in our bodies. Worst of all, the cellular memory doesn't discriminate; it treats everything as literal. It doesn't know that a TV murder wasn't real. Emotional issues are stored memories as well.

DR. BEN SAYS: I don't believe in reincarnation, but I do know that we have cellular memories that come from our ancestors. We get a huge memory download from our parents, grandparents and great-grandparents and on down our ancestral line. So, for example, if some distant ancestor was raped, or committed rape for that matter, that memory is carried forward to you to some extent. It may be diluted by time, but I believe that the water structure around your DNA works like a flash memory and has retained the emotion attached to the lives of our ancestors. You can see how this could be cumulative over time and for some people it is quite overwhelming. With the stress and environmental challenges we're all facing today, it is no wonder that the cancer rates are soaring. That's why it is so important to heal those cellular memories.

Symptoms of breast cancer

Since so many women do their monthly breast self-exams (BSEs) and get clinical breast exams, a large number of suspicious lumps and breast cancers are caught before they cause any symptoms. However, some are not found early enough.

Cancerous lumps are usually hard, painless and with uneven edges, but occasionally they are tender, soft and rounded.

Here are some other signs of breast cancer:

- Lump or mass in the armpit
- A change in the size or shape of the breast
- Abnormal nipple discharge
  Usually bloody or clear-to-yellow or green fluid
  May look like pus
- Change in the color or feel of the skin of the breast, nipple, or areola
  Dimpled, puckered, or scaly
  Retraction, "orange peel" appearance
  Redness
  Accentuated veins on breast surface
- Change in appearance or sensation of the nipple
  Pulled in (retraction), enlargement, or itching
- Breast pain, enlargement, or discomfort on one side only
- Any breast lump, pain, tenderness, or other change in a man
- Symptoms of advanced disease are bone pain, weight loss, swelling of one arm and skin ulceration

If you have been diagnosed with breast cancer

Before we get too far into this subject, we want to offer a few words of caution and encouragement.

The following pages include detailed descriptions of various types of breast cancer and the standard medical approach to their treatment. *Do not read these pages without immediately reading Chapter 11.* If you don't have time to read these two chapters right now, stop and put this book down until you do.

Yes, there is standard medical treatment for all types of cancer and there are many complementary and alternative approaches to breast cancer as well. Remember: You're the one in charge here. You are the one making the decisions. If you've been diagnosed with breast cancer, you owe it to yourself to explore all the options. Your life quite literally may depend on it.

If you've been diagnosed with any type of breast cancer, we understand that this can be a very emotional time for you and your family. Don't try to be stoic. Accept all the love and support that comes your way. It will give you strength. Cry when you need to, celebrate life when you can, take a nap when you need one, eat some chocolate and live every day fully.

You are about to enter a whole new world of cancer terminology and various treatment options. It's not surprising if you are confused.

It is your right to have as much time as you need to get the answers you need to make informed decisions about your treatment. If your oncologist tries to brush you off with a few perfunctory answers in a 10-minute appointment, or rush you or pressure you into making an on the spot decision, then look for a new doctor.

When you go to a doctor's appointment, have a written list of your questions. This way you won't forget a crucial one in the pressure of the moment. When you are provided with answers, take notes. If you don't understand something or your doctor is using words you don't know, don't hesitate to ask for clarification in *plain English*. And take along a friend or relative. Not only will they give you moral support, they'll remember the answers to your questions and probably come up with a few questions of their own.

Types of breast cancer

Ductal carcinoma in situ (DCIS): This is the most common type of breast cancer, accounting for 75 percent of all breast cancer diagnoses. This cancer begins in the cells lining the ducts that bring milk to the nipple. In situ means that the cancer is confined to the milk duct.

Dr. Ben believes that nearly all women over the age of 50 have DCIS. The small number is usually quite harmless until a mammogram machine compresses the duct, causing it to squeeze cells out of the duct and into the tissue where the lymph system can pick it up. Or it becomes dangerous when someone decides to do a biopsy and spreads cells into the lymphatic and circulatory systems.

Sometimes DCIS is described as pre-cancerous, pre-invasive, non-invasive, or intraductal cancer. Some pathologists don't even consider it to be cancer.

Many thousands of women undergo needless surgery, chemotherapy and radiation for DCIS when what is really needed at this stage is prevention, preventing DCIS from developing into invasive breast cancer, the type that has spread to other breast tissue. You already have the tools: an alkaline diet, stress relief, exercise, supplements and addressing cellular memories that compromise your cell structure and your immune system. This, combined with careful watching to make sure the mass is shrinking or at least not growing larger, is appropriate for this type of dysplasia.

If you do decide to have a biopsy – which we do not recommend for DCIS — then here is more information. There are three grades of DCIS: low, intermediate, and high, determined by the way the cells look under a microscope.

The grade relates to how the cells look under the microscope, and gives an idea of how quickly, if ever, the cells will develop into an invasive cancer or how likely it is that the DCIS will come back after surgery. Low-grade DCIS has the lowest risk of developing into an invasive cancer, and high-grade carries the greatest risk.

DCIS is not usually life-threatening. It is non-invasive and is considered the earliest form of cancer, categorized as Stage 0. We'll tell you more about staging later in this chapter. Although this cancer stays inside the milk ducts, having DCIS does increase the risk of an invasive cancer. Most areas of DCIS will never develop into invasive breast cancer even with no treatment. However, standard medicine usually chooses to treat DCIS because it is not currently possible to tell which areas will definitely develop into an invasive cancer.

Lobular carcinoma in situ (LCIS): This condition means there are changes in the cells of the lobules or the milk-secreting glands of the breast. Otherwise, LCIS is fairly similar to DCIS and its risks of spreading are similarly low. Having LCIS does carry a small risk of later developing into invasive breast cancer, but most women with LCIS do not develop breast cancer. The condition is most often found in pre-menopausal women. LCIS is not visible on mammograms or MRIs. However, your thermogram can be very reassuring here if there are no changes reflecting new blood flow patterns. It is usually discovered when a sample of breast tissue is taken and examined under a microscope after a biopsy or when a breast lump is removed.

Invasive breast cancer

These are cancers that have started to break through the normal breast tissue barriers and invade the surrounding areas. Clearly these are far more serious than DCIS or LCIS and require more attention and more aggressive measures.

Some women have what is known as HER2-positive breast cancer. HER2, short for human epidermal growth factor receptor-2, is a gene that helps control cell growth, division, and repair. When cells have too many copies of the HER2 gene, cell growth speeds up. HER2 plays a key role in turning healthy cells into cancerous ones. Some women with breast cancer have too much HER2, and they are therefore considered HER2-positive. Research suggests that women with HER2-positive breast cancer have a more aggressive disease and a higher risk of recurrence than those who have HER2 negative breast cancer.

Infiltrating Ductal Carcinoma (IDC): IDC is the most common type of breast cancer representing 78 percent of all malignancies. On mammograms, these lesions can be star-shaped in appearance or rounded. IDC cells formed in the lining of the milk duct break free of the duct wall and invade the surrounding breast tissue. The cancer cells may stay near their place of origin or they can spread even farther through the body carried by the bloodstream or the lymphatic system.

IDC cancers often have HER2 receptors that require an additional stage of treatment during standard treatment that includes hormone therapy.

Infiltrating Lobular Carcinoma (ILC): This type of cancer is less common than IDC, but it acts in a similar way. ILC starts in the milk-producing lobule and invades the surrounding breast tissue. With ILC, frequently there is no actual lump, but more of a subtle thickening of the tissue and a feeling that the tissue is different from its surrounding tissue. These cancers are difficult to diagnose by mammography. However, it should be obvious as it develops by comparing one thermogram to the next.

Less common types of invasive breast cancer

Inflammatory breast cancer: This is a rare but aggressive type of breast cancer. It may begin as an itchy rash. The skin on the breast becomes red and swollen and may take on a thickened, pitted appearance — similar to an overripe orange peel. This is caused by cancer cells blocking lymph vessels located near the surface of the breast.

Medullary carcinoma: This is a specific type of invasive breast cancer in which the tumor's borders are clearly defined, the cancer cells are large, and immune system cells are present around the border of the tumor.

Mucinous (colloid) carcinoma: With this type of invasive breast cancer, the cancer cells produce mucus and grow into a jelly-like tumor. The prognosis for mucinous carcinoma is better than for other, more common types of invasive breast cancer.

Paget's disease of the breast: This rare type of breast cancer affects the nipple and the dark area of skin surrounding the nipple (areola). It starts in a milk duct, as either an in situ or invasive cancer. If associated with carcinoma in situ, the prognosis is very good.

Tubular carcinoma: This rare type of breast cancer gets its name from the appearance of the cancer cells under a microscope. Though it's an invasive breast cancer, the outlook is even more favorable than it is for invasive ductal carcinoma or invasive lobular carcinoma.

Phylloides tumor: A large, bulky tumor may be an indication of a phylloides tumor, a type of tumor that develops in the connective tissue of the breast, rather than in a duct or lobule. The outlook for a phylloides tumor is uncertain. If the tumor can't be removed, it's difficult to treat.

Metaplastic carcinoma: Metaplastic carcinoma represents less than 1 percent of all newly diagnosed breast cancers. This lesion tends to remain localized and contains several different types of cells that are not typically seen in other forms of breast cancer. Prognosis and treatment is the same as for invasive ductal carcinoma.

Micropapillary carcinoma: This invasive type of breast cancer tends to be relatively aggressive, often spreading to the lymph nodes even when the masses are very small.

Adenoid cystic carcinoma: This type of breast cancer is characterized by a large, local tumor. It's an invasive but slow-growing type of breast cancer that's unlikely to spread.

Stages of breast cancer and their prognosis

All types of cancer are subject to a staging system. This helps you and your doctor know exactly how far advanced the cancer is and what kind of treatment can be most effective. Your doctor may or may not tell you about the prognosis, which is just a fancy term for the expected outcome. This will also give you an idea of the seriousness of the cancer and the survival rates for others with the same degree of cancer spread.

Don't be afraid to ask these questions and to let your doctor know that you can "handle" the answers. Some doctors will try to shield you and your family from the harsh realities if there is a poor prognosis. Kathleen thinks this is unconscionable and in reality robs a person with cancer of the opportunity to live consciously. Yes, we should all live consciously, but few of us do. There is nothing that brings a more bittersweet edge to every breath than knowing each experience, each dawn, each flower blooming, each lover's kiss is to be savored, perhaps for the last time.

Your doctor may give you a five-year survival rate. This is that the percentage of those with the same diagnosis as you have, who are alive five years later. This in no way indicates that you will be well or tumor free. It's just that that percent of people are still breathing at the end of five years. We don't mean to be brutal. It's just that doctors frequently say things in ways that patients don't fully understand and patients don't know the right way to word the question to get a truly helpful answer.

Here are the stages of breast cancer:

Stage 0 usually refers to DCIS or LCIS. These abnormal cells seldom become invasive cancer. However, their presence is a sign that a woman has an increased risk of developing breast cancer. This risk of cancer is increased for both breasts.

Stage I is an early stage of breast cancer in which the cancer has spread beyond the lobe or duct and invaded nearby tissue. Stage I means that the tumor is no more than about an inch across and cancer cells are not believed to have spread beyond the breast.

Stage II is still early stage breast cancer. Stage II means one of the following: the tumor in the breast is less than 1 inch across and the cancer has spread to the lymph nodes under the arm; or the tumor is between 1 and 2 inches (with or without spread to the lymph nodes under the arm); or the tumor is larger than 2 inches but has not spread to the lymph nodes under the arm.

Stage III is also called locally advanced cancer. This stage is divided into two subcategories: Stage IIIa, in which the tumor is larger than five centimeters (two inches) or there is significant involvement of the lymph nodes; Stage IIIb in which a tumor of any size had spread to the skin, chest wall or internal mammary lymph nodes.

In this stage, the tumor in the breast is large (more than 2 inches across) and the cancer has spread to the underarm lymph nodes; or the cancer is extensive in the underarm lymph nodes; or the cancer has spread to lymph nodes near the breastbone or to other tissues near the breast.

Stage IV is metastatic cancer. The cancer has spread beyond the breast and underarm lymph nodes to other parts of the body.

Five Year Survival Rate by Stage

STAGE	SURVIVAL RATE
Stage 0	100%
Stage I	98%
Stage II	88%
Stage IIIA	56%
Stage IIIB	49%
Stage IV	16%

Source: National Cancer Institute

Something else we need to be completely clear about. Let's say you had a Stage II cancer removed. That means there is no cancer in the lymph nodes right? Absolutely wrong! It simply means there are no clusters of cancer cells that the pathologist sees on the slides that he/she is looking at. Individual cells are almost impossible to see. The cluster has to be large enough to catch the pathologist's eye, and the slices of tissue that doctors are looking at could have missed the cancer cells altogether! That's why we encourage you to completely change your lifestyle even if you are told "we got it all".

Standard treatment options

Chapter 11 is all about innovative and effective ways to treat breast cancer. In this section, we're going to briefly introduce you to the options that conventional medicine offers at the various stages of breast cancer and what you can expect if you have been diagnosed with breast cancer. You will decide what to do and when to do it. You may decide to combine some of these therapies with complementary or alternative therapies, as the vast majority of people with cancer do. We want to be sure you have the basics. You can do more research, ask your doctor for options, talk to friends and gather information in whatever way you feel comfortable.

Surgery

Conventional doctors almost always bring in the idea of surgery when there's a diagnosis of any stage of breast cancer, except the very latest stages.

One type of surgery is called a lumpectomy (also known as breast conserving surgery), in which the lump and some tissue surrounding it are removed. Many doctors want to do a procedure called a wide local excision to include surrounding tissue to encompass all affected tissue.

Lumpectomies are often recommended for Stage 0 and Stage 1 cancers.

Partial and radical mastectomies are also options, depending on how large and how far advanced the cancer has become.

A partial mastectomy involves the removal of the entire breast. A radical mastectomy involves the removal of the entire breast, lymph nodes and underlying chest muscle tissue.

Mastectomy is usually recommended in Stage 3 and higher cancers. Stage 2 cancers are a gray area for conventional medicine and sometimes surgeons will recommend mastectomy for Stage 2 cancers that have spread to the lymph nodes. Mastectomy may also be recommended if there is DCIS affecting more than one area of a breast.

With invasive breast cancer, axillary lymph node dissection usually accompanies surgery. This means that an incision is made in the armpit area and around the collarbone area. Some of those lymph nodes are removed and studied to determine if there has been a spread of cancer to these areas.

Surgery is usually an effective means of treating stage I and II cancer. Although there are never any guarantees that the cancer has not spread, it is the best conventional medicine can offer in terms of a "cure."

The risks of surgery are pretty much the same as for other surgeries in terms of the risks of problems with anesthesia and infections.

If the surgeon has done a lymph node dissection, a post surgical risk is arm lymphedema or swelling of the soft tissues in the arm or hand that may be accompanied by numbness, discomfort and sometimes infection. Lymphedema can begin immediately after surgery or it may not occur for years, if ever. The risk of lymphedema is increased if radiation and chemotherapy are added to the treatment regimen. This is an extremely pesky problem.

Dr. Ben doesn't recommend lymph node dissection. Most surgeons these days have scaled back on the radical removal of all axillary nodes because it doesn't change the outcome. However, if your surgeon is recommending lymph node removal, make your wishes crystal clear before the surgery. You can't put lymph nodes back, and lymphedema is a troubling problem to live with.

Radiation

Radiation therapy, also called radiotherapy (a deceptively gentle sounding word), targets cancer cells that may linger after surgery in the area where the lump was removed. The radiation is aimed at a very narrow area to prevent damage to surrounding cells. Women with DCIS are often advised to undergo radiation treatment to reduce their risk of the tumor becoming invasive. The radiation treatment is normally given every weekday for three to six weeks.

Radiation therapy may cause reddening of the skin in the target area. Many women complain of deep fatigue as the course of radiation progresses. All radiation increases the probability of subsequent cancer of the breast as well as other structures in the area such as the thyroid and the lungs.

Chemotherapy

Chemotherapy is called a systemic therapy, which means it is delivered to the entire body through the bloodstream, usually intravenously. It is intended to rid damage of any cancer cells that may have migrated away from the tumor and is usually given in Stage II or higher cancers.

Several types of chemotherapy drugs may be used to interfere with the life cycle of rapidly dividing cancer cells. In order to work, chemotherapy drugs typically damage immune system functions while trying to target the rogue cancer cells. In the process, the body's white cell count is lowered, so anyone undergoing chemotherapy is more susceptible to infection.

While chemotherapy is no picnic (just ask any woman who has endured it!), recent advancements make it far more tolerable than it was just a few years ago.

When you are diagnosed with cancer, it's not just cancer cells that are rapidly dividing in your body. The cells in your blood, mouth, intestinal tract, nose, vagina and hair are also undergoing constant, rapid division, so chemotherapy affects them too, causing unpleasant side effects.

Among the side effects of chemo are nausea, vomiting, diarrhea, fatigue, anemia, numbness in the hands and feet, memory loss, loss of fertility or early induced menopause, loss of taste and smell, mouth sores and last, but far from least, hair loss.

Most breast cancer chemotherapy drugs cause hair loss. For some, this means loss of all body hair. For others, it may mean a dramatic thinning of the hair. The hair will grow back fairly quickly after the chemotherapy treatments are complete. Most women can expect to have about one inch of new hair growth two months after the chemo treatments have ended. Sometimes the hair will grow back in a different color or texture.

Some side effects will dissipate very quickly after treatments end. Others may take longer to correct themselves, and a few may be permanent.

For some people, numbness in the hands and feet remains indefinitely.

Nausea and vomiting usually decrease between treatments and are most noticeable in the two or three days following a treatment, so rearranging schedules to accommodate the need for more rest may be helpful.

Hormonal therapy and targeted therapies

Hormonal therapy is the standard treatment for breast cancer that is hormone-receptor-positive. This is sometimes called "anti-estrogen therapy," since it blocks the ability of the hormone estrogen to turn on and stimulate the growth of breast cancer cells.

For years, Tamoxifen™ was the hormonal medicine of choice for all women with hormone-receptor-positive breast cancer. But in recent years, the results of several major worldwide clinical trials showed that a group of drugs called aromatase inhibitors Arimidex™ (chemical name: anastrozole), Aromasin™ (chemical name: exemestane) and Femara™ (chemical name: letrozole) worked better than Tamoxifen™ in post-menopausal women with hormone-receptive-positive breast cancer.

The current practice is to recommend aromatase inhibitors for post menopausal women with hormone receptor positive breast cancer and Tamoxifen™ for pre-menopausal women. Current recommendations are for women to take these drugs for five to ten years after diagnosis. Among the side effects are early start of menopause, weight gain, mood swings, irritability, depression and hot flashes. For women with metastatic cancer, these drugs can cause burning pain in the bones.

Targeted cancer therapies are cancer treatments that target specific characteristics of cancer cells, such as a certain protein that is part of their makeup, an enzyme that affects the ability of DNA to repair itself or the formation of new blood vessels that feed the tumor. Most targeted therapies are antibodies, so in this way, targeted therapies are very different from more traditional types of anti-cancer therapies.

The major targeted therapies are:

- Herceptin™ (chemical name: trastuzumab), the best known targeted therapy for breast cancer. This intravenous infusion taken once a month works against breast cancers that have extra HER2 genes and make too many HER2 protein receptors. Herceptin™ does have a number of potentially serious side effects, including impaired heart function, infections and lung inflammation plus the hair loss, nausea, diarrhea, fatigue and other side effects commonly associated with chemotherapy.

- Tykerb™ (chemical name: lapatinib) is another targeted therapy that works against very aggressive breast cancers that have extra HER2 genes. The Tykerb™ pill taken once a day has been approved by the FDA to be given in combination with Xeloda™ (chemical name: capecitabine) to treat advanced, HER2-positive breast cancer that has stopped responding to anthracyclines, taxanes and Herceptin. Side effects include generally reversible changes in heart function, shortness of breath, diarrhea, nausea, vomiting, rash and hand-foot syndrome which may include numbness, tingling, redness, swelling and discomfort of the hands and feet.

- Avastin™ (chemical name: bevacizumab) is also a targeted therapy. Avastin™ targets the new blood vessels that feed cancer cells. Avastin™ has been approved by the FDA to treat certain types of advanced cancers of the lung, colon and rectum. Researchers are studying Avastin™ in combination with Taxol™ (chemical name: paclitaxel) to see if the combo can slow the progression of advanced breast cancer better than Taxol™ alone. The side effects associated with Avastin™ are daunting, but this is a drug that is basically a last ditch effort for very advanced breast cancers. Side effects include increased risk of blood clots, extreme high blood pressure, kidney malfunction, vision and nervous system disturbances and gastrointestinal bleeding.

Is a diagnosis of breast cancer a death sentence?

Absolutely not! First of all, it is extremely important that you keep a positive attitude. Knowing what we know about cellular memory and the effects of thought patterns on cells, keeping your thoughts optimistic will make quite important physical differences.

Overall, 86 percent of women diagnosed with all stages of breast cancer will survive for five years. The ten-year survival rate is 76 percent.

For women whose cancers have not metastasized, the five-year survival rate is 96 percent. For women with metastasized breast cancer, the five-year survival rate is just 21 percent.

Between 1976 and 1997, the five-year survival rate increased from 75 percent to 86 percent. This is probably just a statistical skew because we are now detecting cancers that may not be cancer at all, i.e., DCIS and LCIS or at least they would have never been a problem. And of course, if we put these in the statistics as "cures" we are going to look like we have made huge advances when, in fact, breast cancer survival rates for Stage III and IV are virtually unchanged in spite of all of the new extremely expensive drugs.

> ### "DOCTORSPEAK"
>
> Most doctors are in the business of giving hope. That's laudable, but they may not always be giving you the straight story.
>
> For example, when they are attempting to convince you that chemotherapy is the best way to go if you're treating breast cancer of nearly any stage, they'll talk about the chemotherapy agents "shrinking" tumors.
>
> When you hear that the drugs are shrinking tumors, you assume that means the cancer is receding and you think that is a good thing.
>
> Not necessarily. In fact, shrinking tumors means absolutely nothing. Tumor shrinkage is merely a reflection of something that happened in a laboratory, it has nothing to do with what cancerous tumors are doing in your body. Tumor shrinkage has no relationship to life expectancy. We know that sounds a little strange but that's what the numbers show.

If you have been diagnosed with any stage of breast cancer, be strong, but don't be a Superwoman. Accept help, friendship and love. You can be one of the positive statistics if you keep your attitude positive and follow some of the complementary therapies recommended in the next chapter.

Chapter 11 WHAT'S WRONG WITH CONVENTIONAL TREATMENT?

Conventional medical treatment for cancer is almost always a poor choice, with a few exceptions. Chemotherapy drugs and radiation are so toxic in themselves that many patients die of the side effects from the treatment. Others literally starve to death as their bodies become unable to extract nutrients from the food they eat and from the cancer cells' insatiable appetite for sugar.

It's not a pretty picture, but many people don't actually die of the cancer, but from the abuses brought about by well-meaning practitioners of modern medicine.

You've been diagnosed with breast cancer. Now what?

You need the best doctor you can find.

In the best of all worlds, you'd find the ideal oncologist (cancer specialist), preferably one who specializes in women's cancers. This ideal doctor would be completely conversant with and unprejudiced about alternative, integrative and complementary therapies for breast cancer. They're called integrative oncologists and you may find a handful of them in the larger cities. They're kind, caring and dedicated to helping you find a way to heal yourself on all levels, especially freeing you from cancer. They're sort of like Dr. Ben. In fact, they're exactly like Dr. Ben.

Sadly, these doctors are few and far between. Your doctor may be able to refer you to one or find colleagues who can send you in the right direction. The American College for Advancement in Medicine (ACAM) has a doctor finder service at its website: www.acamnet.org or by calling 888-439-6891.

You may have some luck by Googling "integrative cancer specialist" or "integrative oncologist." The best way of all is by word of mouth.

Contact cancer support groups and ask breast cancer survivors about their experiences with integrative specialists. Talk to friends, relatives, co-workers and neighbors. Often the best recommendations come from a friend of a friend.

You, your friends and relatives and anyone else you can recruit, will need to search for the best possible match. You'll all need to educate yourselves and prepare to educate your oncologist.

Your search for the right doctor may be a long struggle, but it is worth the effort. Your life may depend on it.

Conventional doctors know almost nothing about integrative treatments. They only know what they have been taught about treating cancer which is to throw toxic chemicals at it, frequently with little success. Because they are unfamiliar with complementary and alternative medicine (CAM) therapies, they are frequently quite prejudiced against them.

The National Institutes of Health tell us that 93 percent of all cancer patients have used at least one form of alternative therapy, ranging from supplement use to chiropractic, acupuncture, hands on healing, herbals, nutritionals, prayer, meditation and spiritual practices.

Then why are so many doctors so uneducated about the therapies that their patients so clearly are seeking? We don't know the answer, but we hope that more physicians will educate themselves and be willing to think outside of their box. This push will have to come from outside of conventional medicine. That means Dr. Ben, Kathleen and all of you.

Debunking the myth

Surgery can be a cure

Conventional medicine can make few promises, but the best it can give a person with breast cancer is the promise of a cure through surgery.

This may not be true in every case and surgery is not always an option with invasive breast cancers. If the cancer is encapsulated into a manageably-sized tumor and the tumor can be removed without spreading it, a surgical cure is possible.

What's wrong with chemotherapy?

Chemotherapy drugs have several ways in which they attempt to kill cancerous cells, none of them pleasant.

Most of these drugs are designed to kill rapidly dividing cells, and since cancer cells sometimes reproduce more rapidly than other types of cells the idea is that they will kill the cancer.

What really happens is that a good number of the rapidly dividing cells in the body are killed—including those that cause the growth of normal skin cells, hair, nails and those that line the gastrointestinal tract. Worst of all, normally the most rapidly dividing cells in the human body are those of the immune system, so chemotherapy damages the immune system. This makes the patient far more vulnerable to infections, the invasion of other cancers and the growth of the cancer cells the chemo didn't kill.

It's also important to note that chemotherapy drugs do not kill all the cancer cells. At best, they may kill 45, 50 or 60 percent. It's up to your immune system to do the rest of the work and get rid of the remaining invaders. But, since the chemo drugs suppress the immune system, the last cleanup often can't happen. So chemo drugs actually diminish your chances of fighting off the cancer yourself.

This is the place where standard medicine and holistic medicine have a serious parting of the ways. While standard medicine suppresses the immune system, holistic medicine seeks to strengthen the immune system so that the body can naturally fight off cancer, infections and any other invaders or cells that are not behaving properly.

Some anti-cancer drugs attempt to cut off the blood supply to tumors or to induce cancer cells to commit suicide, something called apoptosis, since cancer cells have forgotten that their lifespans must end at some point. These can be useful agents.

The most commonly used chemotherapy drug for breast cancer is doxorubicin (sold under the brand names Adriamycin™, Doxil™, Rubex™). In addition to the fatigue, immune suppression, hair loss and nausea commonly associated with chemotherapy, this drug can cause severe heart damage, sometimes even years after it has been taken. The risk of heart damage is especially high among African-American women. Doxorubicin can also stop the formation of red blood cells in the bone marrow, leading to severe anemia and further compromising the immune system.

Other chemotherapy agents and drugs that are sometimes given after the standard course of treatment is over can cause side effects ranging from extreme dehydration to debilitating bone and joint pain, fluid retention, breathing difficulties, weakening of the heart muscle, interruption of menstrual periods and premature menopause.

One study confirms that some women with breast cancer who receive chemotherapy (in addition to surgery and radiation) had a 28 times greater chance of developing leukemia than those who avoided such drugs.

OK. Let's get a handle on what is really meant by the "improvements" the pharmaceutical industry claims are obtained through chemotherapy. The FDA defines an effective drug as one that achieves a 50 percent or more reduction in tumor size for 28 days. Ralph Moss, PhD, a former science writer and assistant director of public affairs for Memorial Sloan-Kettering Cancer Center, has been an outspoken critic of the cancer establishment. In his book, Questioning Chemotherapy (Equinox Press 1995), Dr. Moss says, "Examining clinical trials, I find that the new drugs do not extend the life of the great majority of adults who receive them. But the public is systematically misled about the value of chemotherapy."

There is no evidence that chemotherapy contributes to the long-term survival of people with advanced breast cancer.

Chemotherapy is not a cure. It doesn't even really delay the progress of cancer or help people with cancer to live longer.

Chemotherapy drugs are toxic and they are outrageously expensive, robbing terminal cancer patients of their quality of life in exchange for a few weeks of life.

Yet those few weeks come at an enormous cost to the human body, quality of life and a patient's pocketbook or, if she's lucky, that of her insurance company.

Exorbitant costs

Recent figures are difficult to find since drug companies guard them so carefully, but it appears that the average single chemotherapy treatment costs $4,500 and, for the average breast cancer patient, eight treatments are administered, plus surgery and radiation. One of the newer drugs costs $20,000 per treatment.

At $8,000 a treatment or more, the company that exclusively markets Taxol™, one of the most commonly used chemotherapy drugs, for years raked in $5 million a day. Not bad, considering Bristol-Meyers Squibb did not develop the drug, the U.S. taxpayers paid for it, and the drug manufacturer managed to gain rights through a protracted court battle. All of this for a drug, that promises nothing but to shrink tumors by 50 percent for 28 days. Remember: Tumor shrinkage does not increase life expectancy.

Just to give you an idea of how outrageously medical costs have escalated, we were able to find some figures on treatment for colon cancer that we think probably parallel those for breast cancer:

The wholesale cost of the drugs used to treat a single colon cancer patient has increased from $500 in 1999 to $250,000 today. Insurers have been willing to pay so far because drugs are still cheaper than surgery.

Stay away from chemotherapy if possible. You may know someone who took the entire standard treatment regimen for breast cancer and survived. We rejoice with you that this is so. She was fortunate. Others are not so fortunate.

Adding insult to injury

In the past few years, oncologists have become enamored with drugs that treat or prevent anemia in cancer patients on chemo. You may have seen the television commercials touting Procrit™, Johnson and Johnson's anemia drug. The others are Aranesp™ and Epogen™ made by Amgen.

The New York Times told us on May 9, 2007 that drug companies pay doctors very large amounts of money to prescribe these essentially useless drugs in large quantities knowing they may provoke heart attacks or strokes.

This is all in the name of big bucks. For example, one group of six cancer doctors (quite legally) received $2.7 million as "incentives" for prescribing $9 million worth of Amgen's anemia products in 2006 alone. In all, hundreds of millions of dollars have been paid to physicians to prescribe these expensive drugs (roughly $200 a dose at the lowest levels; however they are commonly prescribed at very high levels, which costs nearly $7,000 a dose.)

This is so outrageous that we can hardly comment on it. It represents everything that is wrong with conventional medicine.

An FDA (Food and Drug Administration) report says there is no evidence that these medicines have improved the quality of life in patients or have extended their lives. The FDA has suggested it is considering curtailing the use of these drugs in cancer patients.

What's wrong with radiation?

We know radiation causes cancer, so it makes no sense whatsoever to attempt to treat cancer with radiation. It's simply not logical.

DR. BEN SAYS: Radiation increases the speed of oxidative damage to tissues. Oxidative damage is the biological equivalent of rust on a bumper and it leads to all of the degenerative diseases of aging: diabetes, heart disease and – you guessed it – cancer. While oxidative damage is part of the aging process, radiation accelerates that process dramatically. It damages the immune system and increases your risk of a variety of health problems.

Radiation also increases the risk of ploidy. I know that's probably not a familiar word for most of us. Here's what ploidy means to cancer: Cancerous tumors usually have only one cell line. Radiation causes the cell lines to mutate, so where there was once one cell line, after radiation, there might be two, three or even four lines of cancer cells. Now we're fighting not just one but two, three or more cell lines and the cancer's chance of surviving chemo and radiation therapy has increased, while the patient's chance of survival has decreased.

Dr. Ralph Moss, the outspoken critic of conventional cancer care treatment mentioned earlier in this chapter, has some very specific criticisms of radiation therapy:

"Radiation is … a 'perfect carcinogen,' which can both initiate and promote tumor formation. For that reason, I would not be so quick to make adjunctive radiation part of the standard protocol for this precancerous condition (DCIS)."

Dr. Moss went on to say, "I worry about the long-term health effects of radiation therapy. We know, for instance, that in earlier studies of breast cancer, unexpected long-term damage to the cardiovascular and immune systems vitiated any immediate beneficial impact of radiation."

The bottom line: Radiation is not in your best interest for a first line or even a second line treatment. There is a time to use it. We'll talk about it in the next chapter.

Educate yourself

Gone are the days when the doctor made pronouncements and the patients meekly obeyed. Thanks to the Internet, there is an abundance of information on breast cancer, possible CAM (complementary and alternative medicine) treatments and conventional therapies.

It's your responsibility to educate yourself so you can take responsibility for your own health. No one else can or will.

Take the time to learn everything you can. Ask questions of your doctor and form a partnership to find all the right answers for your unique situation.

While there are literally tens of thousands of websites out there, some can be very helpful and others are useless, misleading or even inaccurate. Use your best judgment. If something intuitively seems strange to you, don't pay attention to it. If it speaks to your heart, be sure you've gathered all the information you can and then embrace it.

Chapter 12 CAM THERAPIES FOR BREAST CANCER: A KINDER, GENTLER WAY

There is another way, a kinder, gentler way that enhances your body's inborn healing processes.

No doubt, you've heard of complementary, alternative, and integrative therapies. The terms "complementary" and "integrative" medicine are, for all practical purposes, the same thing. In the research you will inevitably do, you may see the term "CAM," which stands for complementary and alternative medicine. This can encompass anything from vitamins and natural supplements to mystical hands on healing to the principles of quantum physics and *The Healing Codes*™. We'll admit that some of these are pretty far out there in terms of conventional medicine's approach to healing, but given the statistics we gave you in Chapter 10, conventional medicine's approach to cancer hasn't had a very high success rate, so why not stretch out there, take a leap based on good evidence and work with your body for healing?

CAM exists outside the box of conventional medicine. This is because the U.S. government controls that box and the only approved ways to address cancer are surgery, radiation and highly toxic pharmaceuticals including chemotherapy and hormone therapy.

CAM therapies are parallel to standard medical practice. For people undergoing standard cancer treatments, there are many doctors and clinics that offer services that include supplements, nutritional, emotional and spiritual support. One outstanding example of this type of care is the Block Center for Integrative Cancer Care in suburban Chicago. Other outstanding integrative cancer treatments centers include the M.D. Anderson Cancer Center at the University of Texas in Austin and Cancer Treatment Centers of America with four regional centers.

CAM therapies can include the intelligent uses of surgery, chemotherapy and radiation. For example, if a tumor is obstructing a vital vessel such as the spinal cord, aorta, bronchi or common bile duct, radiation can be used as a measure to buy time to let the body get back into balance and perform its own healing. Likewise, there are some progressive doctors who are delivering chemotherapy directly to a tumor by finding the blood vessels that lead into it, putting the drug directly into the vessel and neutralizing the drug as it comes out of the tumor to prevent damage to other tissues. This way, chemotherapy drugs do not harm other parts of the body or weaken the body's natural defense system. In the U.S., this process is called intraarterial chemotherapy. It's called transarterial chemotherapy in Europe. Dr. Ben has sent patients to Mexico for this procedure since the cost is not covered by insurance and it is much less expensive south of the border.

Another intelligent use of pharmaceuticals with which Dr. Ben has had personal experience is IPT or insulin potentiated therapy. This therapy must be administered by someone highly trained and highly skilled in its use, since intravenous insulin is delivered until the patient's blood sugar drops into the 30 to 40 mg/dL range, which is very low. The theory is that by depriving the cancer cells of the sugar that sustains them, the tumor cells will be very open, very hungry, and they will take in small amounts of chemo given while the sugars are so low.

Later in this chapter, we'll talk more about the relationship between cancer and what you eat, but for now, it is very important for you to understand that cancer cells eat sugar. They cannot live on protein or fat, so keeping your diet as low in carbohydrates of all types as possible will help control the cell growth.

The best CAM approaches to breast cancer

No doubt you will be inundated, perhaps overwhelmed with well-meaning advice from friends, family, even strangers, about the best way to treat cancer naturally.

There are some very good cancer treatment plans out there. There are also some really bad ones.

This book would be 1,000 pages long and still missing essential information if we tried to elaborate on every single CAM therapy on the market today.

In addition, every person is unique and individual. You deserve an individually designed treatment plan, so we wouldn't presume to tell you what would be best for you. You and your doctor will make those decisions.

So we've decided to give you what we can on the treatments that specifically relate to breast cancer. These are some of the treatments Dr. Ben found valuable in his integrative cancer practice that included many women with breast cancer:

Electrodermal Screening (EDS)

Electrodermal screening is a great starting place to help you design a course of treatment. EDS uses the principles of Chinese medicine to scientifically track the body's energy meridians that can help you and your doctor design a custom-tailored course of treatment that will work just for you.

The flow of energy (sometimes called chi, ki or prana) along these meridians carries with it information about the internal organs that can be used in arriving at a diagnosis and devising a treatment plan.

The electrodermal screening device works by measuring electrical resistance and polarization at acupuncture points, control measurement points and energy meridians. Through these safe, non-invasive and painless measurements, it is possible to analyze the bio-energy and bio-information produced by internal organs and systems.

What happens in an EDS session? The evaluation is usually conducted by a homeopathic or naturopathic physician, a chiropractor or other trained practitioner.

The patient is asked to hold a stylus with an electrode for grounding purposes in one hand while the doctor presses the tip of a second stylus against the patient's acupuncture points. During the measurement, the patient and the EDS device form a closed circuit, allowing energy and information to flow from the EDS device to the probe, through the patient to the hand electrode, and back to the EDS device. The EDS reading is a measurement of how much energy makes it through the circuit.

Based on a set of pre-determined values, the doctor can identify where there are energetic shortages and then identify substances like herbs, vitamins, minerals and homeopathics that might correct the shortfall.

EDS does not treat cancer. Instead, it gives you and your doctor an idea of which direction to take in your treatment plan. It can help you reject treatments that might not be effective in your particular case and will help point out those that may be the most beneficial.

Homeopathy

We're not going to go into an entire course on homeopathy here, but it bears a few paragraphs of explanation since the theory behind homeopathy is so different from the usual Western concept of medicine.

Homeopathy, discovered by an 18th century German genius named Samuel Hahnemann, is based on the Law of Similars. It's not really much different from the Law of Attraction that we've mentioned many times in this book.

Homeopathy is based on the theory that symptoms are the body's way of fighting disease, so symptoms are to be encouraged with a remedy in minuscule doses that in larger doses would produce the same symptoms seen in the patient. These remedies are meant to stimulate the immune system so the body can heal itself and cure the illness. You may find this theory referred to as "like treating like."

By diluting those symptom-causing agents, mineral or elemental substances in a standardized way, Hahnemann discovered that he could find the true essence of that substance, leading to the understanding of the true essence of the illness in the individual patient. He was actually engaging in quantum physics centuries before the science was discovered by using the energetic signatures of the disease and stimulating the immune system to cure the illness. Hahnemann and his students approached their treatments in a holistic way, dealing with the body, mind and spirit of their patients, not just the symptoms or even the disease.

Classic homeopathic doctors spend extended periods of time with their patients, asking them questions that deal not only with their particular symptoms or illness, but also with the details of their daily lives in order to find the perfect remedy for the entire person.

Nuclear magnetic resonance (NMR) machines have now been used to confirm the subatomic activity in homeopathic remedies, confirming their value as energy medicines.

Homeopathy is now the treatment of choice for 500 million people around the world, including the Queen of England.

This is the barest of explanations of the exceptionally complex science of homeopathy. You can learn more by reading any of Dana Ullman's excellent books on homeopathy or Asa Hershoff's Homeopathic Remedies (Avery 1999) or Miranda Castro's The Complete Homeopathy Handbook (St. Martin's Press, 1990). You'll also find some excellent information and a diagnostic calculator online at www.abchomeopathy.com.

Homeopathy and cancer

It would be tempting to say at this point that you could go out and buy several homeopathic remedies and take them and get rid of your breast cancer. It is not that simple.

First, you will need a homeopathic doctor (naturopaths, N.D.s or N.M.D.s are often well-versed in homeopathy) who can help you devise your own specific remedy that addresses all your symptoms. Electrodermal screening (EDS) is an invaluable tool in helping determine the substances to which your body can best respond. This can also be done with muscle energy testing. It just takes longer.

Homeopathy manipulates the biochemistry and physiology of the human body by using energy rather than physical medicines. When you take a homeopathic remedy, your body recognizes the energy of an extremely dilute substance and uses that energy as a map to help your body move back into perfect balance at the cellular level. This is how homeopathic medicines are used to successfully treat cancer.

Electrodermal screening is a huge step in the right direction, as is blood testing for antibodies to help identify viruses that may be a factor in the cancer in question. Super remedies can be made from this information that will help remove the toxic load, heal the cellular malfunction, heal old emotional wounds (remember *The Healing Codes*™?) and help your body resist the disease.

If you have had a tumor surgically removed, a homeopath can prepare a remedy from the unpreserved tissue. Be sure it is unpreserved since the formaldehyde in which it is usually preserved damages the cells.

A vaccine can also be made by taking a piece of the tumor and culturing it with your white blood cells so that the two work together to teach your immune cells how to make antibodies and the natural killer cells how to seek out and kill these specific tumor cells. This process is illegal in most U.S. states, but many doctors in Japan, China and Germany are making these individualized vaccines.

Frequency devices

Royal Raymond Rife certainly isn't a household name, but he should be celebrated around the world as the man who was able to break the back of cancer all the way back in 1931. This brilliant scientist created an energy frequency generator that could transmit specific electronic signals to destroy living organisms including pathogens, bacteria and cancers. Rife found that by matching the energy signal, frequency or rate of vibration of a cancer cell, the cell would explode from an excess of energy.

In the only study ever performed on Rife's frequency generator, the disease completely disappeared in 14 of 16 people with advanced cancers who had been declared "incurable" by the medical establishment. That study, conducted by a medical team from the University of Southern California, eventually brought about a 100 percent cure rate after the program was adjusted for the remaining two patients.

Rife's work was suppressed, and he and his colleagues castitgated the cancer establishment that was even at that time making billions of dollars a year treating cancer patients.

Today, there are dozens of Rife-inspired devices on the market, but most of them are ineffective because they are not using sufficiently powerful electronic frequencies. Rife's device used megahertz (millions of herz) frequency, exponentially larger than the energy generated in today's devices in the herz range.

"Most of the modern machines do not match the force or the frequency that Rife designed," says Spencer Feldman, a Hawaii-based CAM advocate who is manufacturing a device that does match Rife's specifications. Some CAM practitioners and integrative oncologists have these devices. You can learn more about them at www.rife-machine.com or by calling (888) 456-4268.

DR. BEN SAYS: *In Rife's day, cancer was a much simpler disease. Rife was able to discover the frequencies of the cancer cells and get a 100 percent cure. There is much more cancer today because we all have more emotional overload, informational input and more stress, more toxins, more electromagnetic toxins and just a whole lot more of the "stuff" that causes cancer.*

I think the Rife device was right on the mark. It is one of my fondest dreams to recreate Rife's work and adapt it so it can be effective in the modern world.

Note: Another cancer researcher, Hulda Clark, uses electromagnetic frequencies to treat cancer. While Dr. Ben thinks her work is interesting, he believes she doesn't have the "big picture" because she is blaming most, if not all, cases of cancer on an intestinal parasite. Cancer is a complex disease with many interrelated factors. Clark's approach may be on the right track, but it is far too simplistic.

Natural estriol

When the different types of estrogen occupy the estrogen receptor sites on the cells it's not an all or none phenomenon. Different substances stimulate those receptor sites in various ways. Xenoestrogens are really bad, while the natural estrogen estriol is the least harmful of the estrogens naturally manufactured by the human body. It makes sense to occupy those receptor sites with beneficial estrogens, such as estriol, so there is no space for harmful estrogens to get a toe hold.

If you have breast cancer, Dr. Ben strongly recommends taking estriol to help neutralize the effects of toxic estrogens.

Estriol is available by prescription at compounding pharmacies.

Eat to live

It took until 1984 for the cancer establishment to admit that diet has a role in cancer prevention. They're still refusing to admit that nutrition has a role in cancer treatment.

We're here to tell you they are wrong. Good nutrition has everything to do with cancer prevention and even more to do with cancer treatment.

Cancer is an energy eater. Not only do cancerous tumors thrive on simple sugars, the cancer itself drains your body of its vital force. The body literally begins to cannibalize itself in a voracious search for sugar and nutrients of any type.

For this reason, scientists have in recent years determined that people with cancer need about twice as much protein as the average healthy person. Healthy women need about 50 grams of protein daily, and if you've been diagnosed with cancer, you should aim for 100 grams daily.

The wasting syndrome known as cachexia, in which nutrients are poorly absorbed and the body literally starts consuming muscle tissue and fat in a desperate attempt to survive, is the immediate cause of death in about 40 percent of those who die with cancer.

You do not want to lose weight while you have cancer, regardless of your normal weight status. This is not the time to go on a diet and it is one place where a few extra pounds may serve as a buffer if an imbalance occurs and cachexia sets in. If you begin to lose weight, speak to your doctor about it immediately.

Eat high quality proteins in organic eggs, lean red meats, poultry and wild-caught fish.

Whey protein

Whey is an excellent source of protein and it's an easy way to boost your protein intake. Whey is that thin watery liquid that rises to the top of your yogurt container. It's a byproduct of milk. Body builders use whey protein to bulk up their muscles and you'll have a similar purpose when you add this tasteless powder to shakes, sauces, cereals and soups.

As with serious athletes, cancer patients often have reduced glutathione levels and a weakened immune system. Numerous studies have shown that whey protein, rich in the amino acid cysteine, provides an extra boost to the immune system by raising glutathione levels. This may help reduce the risk of infection and improve the ability of the immune system to respond to invaders like cancer cells.

Whey protein and cysteine may have some specific benefits for women with breast cancer. At the 2003 annual meeting of the American Cancer Society, research was presented showing that women with the highest levels of plasma cysteine had a 56 percent reduction in the risk of breast cancer compared to individuals with the lowest levels of plasma cysteine. An earlier U.S. Department of Agriculture study had shown similar preventive effects of whey protein.

Because most whey protein products have the lactose removed, they are acceptable for people with lactose intolerance.

When you're choosing a whey protein product, look for one that is unflavored so it can be added to anything. There are hundreds of products on the market, so be a careful label reader. Ideally, you'll want an organic product that is low temperature processed to preserve the delicate amino acids, especially the cysteine. Avoid any products that have added sugars, artificial flavorings or fats. Some milk shake-like whey products are sweetened with stevia, an acceptable and healthy sweetener, if you decide to go for a flavored form.

Dietary recommendations

If you have cancer, you need to eat a high energy diet rich in the most life-promoting foods possible.

This almost always means you should go organic. Think of these life-affirming foods as your prescription for recovering your health. Re-read Chapter 4 and the recommendations made for a breast healthy alkaline diet. There is no time like the present to commit yourself to changing your internal environment that has supported the growth of cancer cells. Choose now to eat right and stop cancer growth.

You may have to do some experimentation to find what's effective and what makes you comfortable.

There are those who strongly advocate a macrobiotic diet, the Japanese-style diet that is heavy on brown rice and pickled vegetables.

Proponents of macrobiotics say that cancer cannot grow in a body nourished in this way. That's not necessarily true. Objective analysis says that 15 to 20 percent of people with cancer are able to improve their condition through macrobiotics. This may not seem like a great improvement, but consider that most people who turn to macrobiotics to help treat their advanced cancers have run out of conventional therapies. If you want to try macrobiotics, go for it. Start as early as possible.

Dr. Ben highly recommends the detoxification program recommended by noted cancer specialist John Diamond, M.D.

Dr. Diamond's program is based on the theory that accumulated toxins in the body suppress the immune system and promote the growth of cancer cells. He recommends avoiding toxins whenever possible, in air, food and water.

Then he calls for an aggressive program to shore up the defenses of the major organ systems involved in detoxification: colon, liver, kidneys, the lymphatic system and skin.

The intestines are an especially important part of the Diamond detoxification program because they contain more lymphoid immune tissue than any other organ. Bowel health is best restored with a high-fiber, low-fat diet, using homeopathics like nux vomicus, berberis homacord and Hepeel™. Probiotic supplements help support beneficial bacteria in the digestive tract.

CO2 (carbon dioxide) therapy

You know the benefits of an alkaline diet. Carbon dioxide therapy goes a step further: By inhaling carbon dioxide, you can alkalinize your blood, further deterring the development and growth of cancer cells. Remember that an acid environment is one of the primary causes of cancer? Alkalizing your body is a matter of pushing the oxygen-hemoglobin disassociation curve in the other direction. Carbon dioxide or CO2 pushes your internal environment toward the alkaline side. It is absolutely the easiest and fastest way to achieve alkalinity. Dr. Ben swears by CO2 therapy – and he's tried everything!

Tips for happier and healthier eating

These eating tips may help reduce the uncomfortable symptoms that accompany cancer:

- Eliminate foods that are common allergens including dairy products, wheat gluten, soy, corn, preservatives and chemical food additives. You may want to be tested for food allergies.

- Eat lots of food high in B-vitamins, calcium and iron, including almonds, beans, whole grains, dark leafy greens and sea vegetables.

- Eat cruciferous vegetables like broccoli, cabbage, cauliflower and Brussels sprouts. They contain numerous anti-cancer nutrients.

- Eat foods high in disease-busting antioxidants, including blueberries, cherries, pomegranates, tomatoes, bell peppers, onions and garlic.

Supplements

We talked about supplements for breast health in Chapter 3. All of these are helpful for breast health and for wellness if you have been diagnosed with cancer, so you might want to re-read that chapter and add some of these to your regimen.

Of course, you're taking routine supplements like multi-vitamins, basic minerals like calcium, magnesium, zinc and selenium and your Omega-3 fatty acids, right? You'll keep on taking these, but consider adding some of the following supplements that have been shown to be specifically helpful in treating cancer, enhancing immune system function and assisting with detoxification.

Remember that the human body has its cycles and when you are taking these supplements (and herbs), with most of them, you'll get better results if you take them for a few weeks and give yourself a break for at least week before you resume taking them. The other option would be to take your supplements Monday through Friday with weekends off.

Talk this over with your doctor and find the supplements that are most appropriate for you:

Cesium: This little-known mineral has a unique electrical charge on every molecule. Unlike normal cells, cancer cells have a very low electrical voltage that allows only five substances to pass into the cell unassisted: water, sugar, potassium, cesium and rubidium. We know that sugar feeds the cancer's growth, but cesium is an extremely alkaline mineral, so it kills the cancer cell.

Recommended dosage: 3 grams daily in divided doses of 1 gram per meal, taken with food. Cesium can be slightly nauseating so it must be taken with food. Many physicians prescribe much higher doses, but you would need to be under the care of a physician and getting routine lab work for higher dosages.

CoQ10: If you're not taking Coenzyme Q10, it's time to start. The National Cancer Institute says that some people with cancer, including breast cancer, have low levels of CoQ10 in their blood. Among CoQ10's many functions is its ability to enhance immune function.

Recommended dosage: 200 mg daily.

Ellagic acid: This powerful antioxidant found in fruits, berries and some nuts has been shown to stop DNA damage that leads to cells mutating into cancer. It stops tumor growth and causes normal cell death among those cancer cells that would like to be immortal. Ellagic acid is usually not taken alone, but as part of a nutritional regimen for cancer treatment, however supplements are available. Eat all sorts of berries, especially red raspberries and grapes and walnuts to get more ellagic acid.

Recommended dosage for cancer patients: 6 grams daily.

L-Lycine and L-proline: For a cancerous tumor to grow, it secretes substances that actually dissolve the nearby tissues in order for it to have space to expand. These two unique proteins stop the dissolving process so tumors have no room to grow. It should be available in any well-stocked nutrition shop.

Recommended dosage for cancer patients: 500 mg of each, three times a day.

Melatonin: This hormone regulates your body's natural sleep-wake cycles and suppresses the production of excessive amounts of sex hormones, which makes it important for anyone with breast cancer who wants to keep estrogen production at a low level. Research also shows that people with breast cancer have low melatonin levels.

Recommended dosage: The dosage used in studies was 20 mg daily, but this is very high. Be sure to use melatonin at these levels only under medical supervision.

Pycnogenol: This substance made from the bark of a particular type of pine tree is one of the most powerful substances known that can selectively target and kill breast cancer cells. Pycnogenol is a strong antioxidant.

Recommended dosage: up to 300 mg daily.

Tetrathiomolybdate: Copper is essential to the formation of blood vessels that supply cancerous tumors. Tetrathiomolybdate binds itself to the copper in order to stop the new blood vessel growth, thereby depriving the tumors of their nutrient supply.

Recommended dosage for cancer patients: 120 mg a day. This has recently been approved as a drug, so you'll need a prescription for it, although you may still be able to find it on the Internet.

Herbs

Bitter Melon (Momordica charantia): Early studies suggest that one of the components of bitter melon extract may be effective in slowing the growth or spread of some types of cancer, particularly breast cancer. Bitter melon also spurs natural tumor-killing cells to perform better and increase their numbers faster so they can seek out and destroy cancer cells.

Recommended dosage: Up to six tablespoons of liquid juice daily. Bitter melon is sometimes injected by a physician.

Essiac tea: This tea, made of burdock root (Arctium lappa), wild sheep sorrel (Rumex acetosella), slippery elm (Ulmus fulva) and turkey rhubarb (Rheum palmatum) is a very popular remedy for cancer, although it has never been scientifically validated. Anecdotal evidence gives this Native American traditional remedy a high potential and many cancer patients say they owe their lives to its abilities to strengthen the immune system and actually flush tumors out of the body. While Essiac tea can be bought in liquid extracts (and in pill form and tea bags, which most practitioners consider worthless), some recommend brewing your own mixture and infusing it with your personal energy. Watercress (Nasturtium officinale R.Br.), blessed thistle (Cnicus benedictus L.), red clover (Trifolium pratense L.), and kelp (Laminaria digitata [Hudson] Lamx.) have been added to later recipes for a product sold as Flor Essence™.

Recommended dosage for cancer patients: At least 1 oz. three times daily.

KATHLEEN SAYS: *My friend Gisela swears that Essiac tea saved her life 15 years ago after her diagnosis with Stage 4 ovarian cancer. Doctors could find no signs of cancer about a year after she started taking the formula, which at the time was available almost clandestinely by mail order from Canada. We know there is no scientific evidence for the effectiveness of Essiac tea, but millions of cancer survivors attribute their healing to this tea. If it's a placebo effect, it's a huge one! Gisela was in her early 30s at the time of her diagnosis and she has continued to drink Essiac tea daily and says she will do so for the rest of her life. We hope it's a long one!*

Graviola (Annona muricata) also known as Brazilian paw paw: For more than 30 years, the National Cancer Institute has known about graviola's ability to kill and selectively target malignant cells of 12 different types of cancer, including breast cancer, without harming healthy cells. One study showed that graviola was 10,000 times more effective in killing colon cancer cells that Adriamycin™, the leading chemotherapy agent. Graviola is a keystone in Dr. Ben's cancer treatment plan.

Recommended dosage: In tincture form, take one teaspoon three times a day or, in pill form, 500 mg a day.

Green tea: Dozens of scientific studies confirm the antioxidants and anti-cancer properties of green tea. The major cancer preventers are antioxidants epigallocatechinallate (EGCG) and epigallocatechin (EGC), close molecular cousins to other flavonoids found in broccoli, cabbage, grapes and red wine that are known to help prevent cancer. More recently, scientists have found that green tea has a unique ability to reverse the genetic damage caused by environmental toxins, particularly turning off the cancer gene that cigarette smoke turns on.

Recommended dosage: If you're drinking it as a tea, drink as many cups daily as you like. Green tea does have caffeine, so you might want to seek out a decaffeinated product. It's also available as an extract in pill form. If you choose a pill form, you'll want 500 mg daily or more.

Hoxsey Remedy: This herbal formula has been around since the 1920s, and it's another with no scientific validation, but exceptionally loyal followers who swear by its ability to remove toxins, strengthen the immune system, enhance the ability to destroy tumors. The developer of the formula, Harry Hoxsey, was endlessly persecuted by the government, the courts, the press and the medical establishment. The Hoxsey formula is illegal in the U.S., but is offered at a clinic in Mexico that is still run under Hoxsey's name. Hoxsey formula is used in two parts, a tonic taken internally and a salve used externally. The brown tonic contains a mixture of supplements and herbs that includes pokeweed, burdock root, licorice, barberry, buckthorn bark, stillingia root, red clover, prickly ash bark, potassium iodide and cascara. The salve includes antimony trisulfide, zinc chloride, blood root and a yellow powder consisting of arsenic sulfide, sulfur and talc.

Recommended dosage: Take as directed.

Milk thistle (Silybum marianum): This prickly herb helps strengthen the liver and aids in the detoxification process, an essential part of cancer therapy. The National Cancer Institute cites research that recommends silymarin, one of the active ingredients in milk thistle, for its ability to stop the growth of certain types of cancer cells. The NCI also says silymarin may enhance the effectiveness of chemotherapy.

Recommended dosage for cancer patients: Up to 160 mg three times daily.

Mushroom extracts: The immune-boosting powers of several types of mushrooms are well-documented. Shitake, maitake and reishi mushrooms are able to enhance the production of natural killer (NK) cells, the immune system's Super Ninja cancer killing cells. There are several good mushroom products on the market, including one that is superextracted called AHCC™. Another mushroom product, MGN-3™, is fairly expensive (about $300 a month for the first two months, then the dosage is lowered), but it begins increasing NK cell production within a week and boosts it by 300 percent until you stop taking it. Consider MGN-3 if you have an invasive Stage 3 or higher cancer.

Recommended dosage: Follow manufacturers' instructions, since each product is very different. It is important to use the recommended dosage for cancer treatment, since it will likely be higher than normal usage.

Sangre de drago (Croton lechleri) also known as dragon's blood: This legendary antioxidant comes from the sap of an Amazon rainforest tree, which contains nearly astronomical quantities of proanthocyanadins, the antioxidants that make red wine so healthful. It is also an antiviral, addressing the viral infections Dr. Ben has found affect virtually every cancer patient. It has also been shown to selectively target and kill cancer cells; and works against viral infections, which we know have a role in cancer.

Recommended dosage: 500 mg four times daily.

Una de gato or cat's claw (*Uncaria tomentosa*): Antiviral action has recently been confirmed in this rain forest herb, and since we know that viruses play a key role in causing cancer, its effects are probably related to the ability to kill viruses and stimulate the immune system.

Recommended dosage: 20 mg three times a day, in tincture 10-15 drops.

DR. BEN SAYS: Immune stimulants should not be taken on a non-stop basis. However, most patients and many doctors aren't aware of this. Everything in nature cycles! You cannot stimulate the immune system endlessly. You must give it breaks, whether it is taking weekends off or three weeks on and one week off.

Lifestyle

Everything about your lifestyle has brought you to the place where you are and everything about it can relieve you from that toxic place and bring you back to health.

Support

If you have breast cancer, the more support you have, the better your outcome will be. Cancer survival improves greatly if a woman feels nurtured and her emotional state is more calm and relaxed, she's focused on the positive and she is able to manage stress.

Having friends around to laugh with you and cry with you is essential. Be sure to ask for and accept lots of hugs.

Your spouse may be less able to deal with his own emotional response to your diagnosis, so help from friends and family is essential for him, too.

Join a support group. Learn to ask for help and to accept help when it is offered.

By the way, a dog or a cat is a wonderful companion and supporter. Just petting a dog or hugging a cat will most definitely ease your physical and emotional pain.

KATHLEEN SAYS: Twenty years ago, when my cousins Mary and Ann were diagnosed with breast cancer, Mary's twin sister, Marty, just waited for the other shoe to drop. Their mother, my aunt, had died of breast cancer a few years before and all three sisters were terrified.

Then, six years ago, came the day Marty had dreaded: she had Stage 2 breast cancer. Because I live closest to her, I was honored to help Marty through her terrible journey.

From the lumpectomy to the grueling chemo sessions and the exhausting daily radiation treatments, Marty was a trooper. She only missed two days of work, a 90-minute drive from her home, through the entire ordeal. I am happy to say that today, six years later, having survived chemo and radiation, she is relatively healthy and enjoying a new career as an award-winning artist.

As I watched Marty struggle with her diagnosis and her treatment, I realized that there were times that she needed a friend and a shoulder to cry on.

There was the sunny Sunday afternoon when Marty, Mary and I declared that we would not allow cancer to control us and ceremonially shaved Marty's head before the chemo drugs could do the job for her.

There were the times when she was so sick after chemo treatments that she'd need to nap on my couch before continuing her 45-minute drive onward to her home.

There was the hilarious hat party night when a large group of friends got together to adorn Marty's beautifully bald pate with silly hats, serious hats and loving poetry.

There were the times when she was so exhausted she couldn't fight with the dastardly insurance company that didn't want to give her the expensive anti-nausea drugs prescribed by her oncologist.

I couldn't take away her pain and fear, but I could be there for Marty. I could be her champion when she needed me or just give her a cup of tea and leave her alone when she needed that, too. I am deeply grateful Marty is still here and plans to be here for a long time.

While I was repulsed by the destruction conventional medicine had brought upon the woman I regard as a sister, I honored the choice of treatment she had made.

And I came to realize that every cancer patient needs a support structure. She needs advocates, friends, cheerleaders, and willing hands to take over the housework when it is just too much. She needs fellow survivors who have walked the same road she is walking and can encourage her along the way.

If you or someone you love has breast cancer, remember that support is more than half the battle.

The spiritual life

Whether or not you look to a Higher Power, your spiritual life is a key part of bringing your body mind and spirit back into alignment, healing those toxic cellular memories and making you whole again.

Whether you use meditation, prayer or both, it will make a difference. Prayer is about asking for things, and it should not be all about you. Meditation is about listening for answers, or just listening and being still. What is important is that you take time to be with yourself, to be in silence and to find solace in the silence and seek the wisdom to hear the answers when they are offered.

Exercise

We've already addressed the importan of exercise. If you have cancer, you may have difficulty finding the energy to exercise. However, researchers have found that women with breast cancer who exercise find that the physical activity actually increases their energy levels.

Yoga, chi gong and tai chi are all gentle, yet powerful forms of exercise that will give you all the benefits of exercise and help you with some of the spiritual aspects of your life as well. Swimming is wonderful exercise and increases lymphatic drainage too.

Massage

Massage may sound like a luxury, but it is an important part of cancer treatment because it will help move the toxins out of your system through the lymphatic system.

Look for a massage therapist who is comfortable with massaging someone with cancer. Most massage therapists are taught that massaging cancer patients might dislodge the cancer and cause it to spread.

Nothing could be further from the truth. Gentle, but firm massage will stimulate lymph flow and help with the healing process.

If you are comfortable with the idea, it is helpful to have your massage therapist include your breasts in the massage treatment. If that is distressing to you, learn to do your own breast massage and perform it daily.

In conclusion...

This chapter represents the barest tip of the iceberg when it comes to CAM therapies for breast cancer. These are simply some of the therapies Dr. Ben has found to be effective for the largest percentage of his patients.

If you are interested in a therapy that is not mentioned here or if you're interested in one of these and want more information, take the time to educate yourself. Ask your health care practitioner to join you in the research. Make wise choices and choose life.

Chapter 13 FEARING THE RETURN OF THE BEAST

If you've had cancer, if someone you love has had cancer or if you're at high risk for cancer, you can guess what we're going to say: The Beast is not the cancer. The Beast is how you think about cancer.

We've talked about the Law of Attraction throughout this book, so you have a good, solid foundation in the power of your mind, emotions and past experiences to mold who you are today and what is happening in our life.

So you've survived cancer. What do you think will happen if you allow yourself to be consumed with the fear that that cancer will return?

You may recall that earlier in this book we mentioned that people who fear cancer most tend to be the ones who get it. This is not some genetic predisposition or mystical bad juju. It's because our minds and even our cellular memories are affected by the fixation on cancer, so fearing cancer creates the perfect toxic environment to bring cancer into your life.

Kathleen believes that the subconscious mind does not comprehend negatives. For example, if your mind is continuously chanting the mantra, "I don't want my cancer to return," your subconscious mind (and every single cell in your being) hears instead, "Cancer, cancer, cancer" or worse yet, "My cancer, my cancer, my cancer...."

On some subtle level, those thoughts begin to imprint themselves upon your cells and change your universe, so that you get cancer.

Obviously you don't want cancer and you don't want cancer to return if you've had it, so you can choose health, wholeness and vitality. Cancer doesn't have to be part of your vocabulary or part of your mental state. You're done with cancer and cancer is done with you. Remember?

This is where *The Healing Codes*™ come in. Practice the breast health code we gave you in Chapter 7 and know that remnants of ancient cellular memories are being healed every time you do this. Your thoughts and your actions will make all the difference in the world. The most important thing you will do for the remainder of your life is to keep yourself emotionally clear.

Chances of recurring breast cancer

We told you in Chapter 10 that, if you have been diagnosed with breast cancer, it is very likely that individual cancer cells have already spread to other parts of your body. Your job now is not to focus on those cells, but to focus on changing permanently the environment and circumstances that allowed that cancer to form in the first place.

Dr. Ben offers what seems like a paradox here: eat, exercise and live in the physical realm as though those cells have metastasized. Emotionally keep yourself completely clear and choose a lifestyle that nurtures wellness. Live in love and forgiveness with everyone!

If that sounds confusing, it's really not.

We all have literally thousands of emotional issues that have created the toxic environment in our bodies that allowed cancer to get a foothold.

It is entirely possible that cancer will recur. It does in many women who have been diagnosed with all stages of breast cancer. In this chapter, we'll go over some health behaviors that will reduce those risks substantially. If the cancer does come back, pick yourself up, dust yourself off and start your cellular health process all over again.

Here's the kicker: You have created an environment in your body that allowed cancer to form in the first place. Now it is your job to change that environment.

Whoa! Stop right now. Is your mind whirling with feelings of guilt?

"Oh, me, poor me, I made myself get cancer. I'm such a bad person." Sniff. Sniff.

Don't go there! That's the most destructive type of thinking you can possibly engage in. Feeling guilty, feeling victimized, feeling sorry for yourself are all ways to create more toxicity in your environment and increase your risk that 'The Beast' will return.

It's quite literally time to change your life. Stand in your power. It takes courage to defeat cancer. Now is the time to live your life in love, not in fear.

Create a friendly, healthy environment and live in it.

How do you do that?

Clean up your act

If you're not already squeaky clean, there's no better time than now to get that way. Some of this is repetitive for a reason: We want to be sure you get the message.

Don't smoke. If you smoke, stop. Today! You've been given a second lease on life. Don't mess it up with the single most destructive habit you could possibly have. Smoking increases your risk of breast cancer, it increases your risk that breast cancer will return and it puts all of those around you at risk.

Limit alcohol consumption. If you drink alcohol, limit your consumption to one drink a day or less. A drink is defined as 5 ounces of wine, 12 ounces of beer or 1 ounce of hard liquor.

Get the lard out. That means get out there and do some vigorous exercise for at least 30 minutes a day, an hour a day if you canmanage it. Whatever exercise you really enjoy will go a long way toward keeping you healthy.

Ditch the plastic. Don't eat or drink out of plastic containers. Don't use them for cooking—especially in a microwave since they are full of cancer-causing xenoestrogens. This includes Styrofoam.

Go organic in your lawn and garden. Don't keep pesticides and herbicides around your house. Don't use them on your lawn or gardens. Not only are they toxic when they are applied, you are likely to carry them into the house on your shoes and leave the toxic chemicals on the floors where babies crawl and pets lie. These chemicals remain toxic in the soil and in your house for years.

Rid your environment of toxic metals. We live in a metallic world. It's nearly impossible to avoid touching metal keys, doorknobs, tools or to avoid drinking water from copper pipes, getting mercury amalgam dental fillings or eating food cooked or food stored in aluminum or metal containers, but be conscious and avoid toxic metals as much as you can. Take some liposome encapsulated EDTA to help get out the metals already in your body.

Refuse all X-rays. Unless they are absolutely essential, say no to all X-rays because they are sources of cancer-causing radiation. This includes CT scans and especially mammograms, which emit approximately 1,000 times the amount of radiation as the average chest X-ray. Ultrasound, MRIs and thermography are better options.

Ditch your TV. The vast majority of what's on television negatively impacts our cellular memories. Just a reminder: If you watch a shoot 'em up on television, your cells don't differentiate that from witnessing an actual murder, so the cellular memory of that violence will be with you (and your descendants) for a very long time. Monitor carefully what you and your family watch on TV. TV is a huge part of our toxic environment.

Practice safe sex. There is a distinct link between viral load and all types of cancer. The three viruses most often detected in people with cancer are all transmitted through body fluids, either orally or sexually. Use discrimination when choosing your partner and always use a condom unless you have been in a monogamous relationship for more than one year with a person you absolutely trust and who has tested negative for sexually transmitted diseases.

Eat healthy food

This means your diet should be rich in whole foods: organic fruits, vegetables, nuts, grains, lean meats and healthy oils. It should be prepared with love and thoughts of healing.

We've said it all before, but it bears repeating in brief. Re-read Chapter 4 for details:

- Avoid all processed foods, soft drinks, white breads, white rice and pasta.
- Banish table sugars from your life. Ditto for pastries, donuts and other high-sugar foods as well as products containing corn syrup.
- Avoid canned foods (except tomatoes and beans), because they are devoid of nutrition.
- Eat organic as much as possible.
- Buy local food. It's fresher and has more nutrients.
- Plant a garden. The exercise will do you good, and you'll get the freshest food possible.
- If you cannot buy organic meats and dairy products, cut your meat and dairy consumption in half.
- Eat the leanest meats possible.
- Eat a wide variety of foods to take advantage of the unique nutrients in each one.
- Drinks lots of pure water.

- Follow an alkaline diet that emphasizes fruits, vegetables and whole grains to create an environment that is inhospitable to cancer.

Plan for long-term health

Life after cancer is much the same as life to prevent cancer.

Somewhere along the line, many of us got the idea that we could get healthy by jogging for 20 minutes on Sunday or eating vegetarian once a month or taking a multi-vitamin when we remember it.

It simply doesn't work that way. Health is a lifestyle. It is a lifetime commitment to take care of the precious temple in which we dwell and which we want to serve us well into the future.

Health means:

- *Supplements:* Take the best ones every day. Take a great multi-vitamin and breast health supplements along with whatever other ones work best for you.

- *Thermograms, not mammograms:* Get an annual thermogram or more often if your doctor so recommends. If you've had breast cancer, you might consider having a whole body thermogram that could point out potential trouble spots outside of your breasts long before they become dangerous. Avoid mammograms at all costs because they brutally compress delicate breast tissue, increasing the risk of dislodging cancer cells if they are present and because a single mammogram delivers the same amount of cancer-causing radiation as if you had 1,000 chest X-rays. The accumulated mammogram radiation from 20 or 30 years of radiation makes it no surprise that older women have a much higher risk of breast cancer than younger women.

- *Blood tests:* If you've had breast cancer, certain markers in your blood can indicate the return of cancer. Regular testing (every six months or so) can re-assure you and give you a heads up if 'The Beast' is re-awakening. As body cells die at the end of their natural life cycle, their contents dissolve and they are scavenged by the lymphatic system and carried through the blood. These tests are looking for little pieces of those cells in the blood that are identifiable as tumor markers. Probably the best blood test and the most accurate one for people in early stages of breast cancer is the AMAS (Anti-Malignan Antibody in Serum) test. It is a relatively new one that measures specific blood antibodies (proteins in the blood that help the body fight disease) called malignans. Malignan antibody levels are higher in people with early stage breast cancer so this blood test can be helpful in early detection. AMAS can also be helpful in determining the return of cancer once treatment is complete. Research showed that in control groups of women with known breast cancer, the test was 96 percent accurate. You should also follow any tumor marker that has shown up during regular blood tests. Your doctor should have told you if you have one of these – but it never hurts to ask just in case the information wasn't passed on.

- *Chelation:* Most of us have accumulated a junkyard of heavy metals in our bodies over a lifetime. Toxic substances like mercury, lead, arsenic, beryllium, cadmium, copper, iron and nickel are ever present in our environment. We breathe them in, we eat them, we even wear them on cotton clothing made from crops saturated in pesticides and then we absorb them through our skin. These heavy metals damage DNA and cause cancer. Get tested and seek out the best possible treatment. The only supplement that has much effect is chlorella. Usually, a special formula of EDTA encapsulated in liposomes called chelation therapy is the best way to usher these toxins out of your body.

- *Have mercury amalgam fillings removed:* The presence of toxic amalgam fillings in your body, shedding mercury molecules with every bite you take, is a major contributor to your toxic environment. If you have mercury amalgam fillings, have them removed by a competent dentist who knows how to do so without spilling more toxins into your body. Look for a mercury-savvy dentist at The Dental Wellness Institute's website, http://www.dentalwellness4u.com.

De-stress your life

That's probably the most difficult task we have placed before you, but it's also the most important. Stress neutralizes all of our good intentions and all of our hard work. Take this seriously.

- *Slow down.* Everything doesn't have to be finished today. Leave the dirty dishes in the sink and take time to talk to your spouse instead. Let the whole family chop up veggies for a huge dinner salad rather than preparing an elaborate meal. Let your kids have a summer to simply be kids rather than planning activities for every waking moment. Learn to say "no" when you're asked to take on a new responsibility. You'll all be happier and healthier.

- *Media fast:* Turn off the TV, the computer, cell phones, unplug the phone and spend a quiet day with family, reading or enjoying nature. Try this once a week. It may become addictive!

- *Breathe:* Yoga teaches us that mind and breath are intimately connected. Deep slow breathing calms racing thoughts, slows the fight-or-flight response, energizes you when fatigue sets in and even cures insomnia. Try sitting quietly for five minutes, taking deep, slow breaths through your nose, at least twice a day.

- *Laugh:* Laughter is one of the greatest stress relievers ever. It not only brings oxygen to your system, it actually reduces levels of the stress hormone, cortisol and, best of all, improves your immune system's ability to produce disease-fighting warrior cells. So rent some old Marx Brothers or Three Stooges movies and laugh yourself healthy several times a week.

Create a strong social and family circle

Whether you are sick or vibrantly healthy, medical science is just starting to realize the power of the link between a strong support network of family and friends and your physical, emotional, mental and spiritual health.

If you don't have a spouse, partner or close friend living in your home, ask yourself, "Why not?" Are you closed to relationship and love? It won't happen overnight, but open yourself to finding the perfect relationship. Think about becoming the type of person you would like to attract into your life. Use the Law of Attraction and what you seek will come.

A close circle of friends is the next best thing. Getting together frequently, sharing a cup of tea, a laugh, a brisk morning walk, all of these things actually strengthen our immune systems and keep us healthy.

Part of the benefit stems from devoting yourself to someone else. If you don't have that close circle, start forming one.

Look at your interests and volunteer somewhere that will be fulfilling, whether it's the local animal shelter, a day care center, church or a nursing home. You'll find like-minded people, fulfilling work and growing relationships with new friends.

Spiritual life is important

It matters what you believe, but maybe more important to your health is that you believe something. We wouldn't presume to tell you what to believe, but choosing a spiritual path not only gives you an anchor in life and a path to walk, it actually contributes to longer life. A University of Pittsburgh study actually showed that people who go to church every week add an average of three years to their lives.

Prayer and meditation are the hallmarks of most religions, as are charitable works, family and a community of like-minded people.

Find a spiritual path, plant your feet firmly upon it and your life will change in ways you cannot imagine.

In conclusion...

None of us knows how many days are left to us on this earth. Whether your time is short or long isn't really the issue. What matters is that you live the happiest life you can possibly create for yourself. What matters is living a life of love and service. What matters is reveling in the abundant sheer joy of life, and when it is time to go on to the next world, to die knowing, however small your contribution might seem, that your life changed the world.

Dr. Ben's parting words to you are a mantra of long life, love and joy that all women can adopt:

I'm going to live to be 120 years old, and die in my lover's arms with both breasts intact.

GLOSSARY OF TERMS

Antigen: A molecule that triggers the immune response and causes the formation of antibodies.

Antibodies: Proteins in the blood that help the body fight bacteria, fungi, and viruses.

Areola: The skin around the nipple that is slightly darker in color than the rest of the breast.

Breast abscess: An area of the breast that has become infected and filled with pus. A breast abscess looks like a hard breast lump that is red, tender, and painful.

Breast cyst: A closed sac or pouch, sometimes found in the breast(s), that contains fluid (part liquid and part solid) or a solid material.

Breast duct: Breast tissue contains many milk ducts, which are small tubes used to transport fluids through the breast. When a woman is breast feeding, milk travels through the dilated (widened) milk ducts in her breasts and out through a small hole in her nipple.

Carcinoma: A solid tissue cancer as opposed to a blood cancer like leukemia.

DCIS: Ductal carcinoma in situ.

Estrogen: The major female hormone, which is composed of three predominant hormones: estriol, estradiol and estrone.

Estrogen dominance: The state when there is insufficient progesterone to balance the estrogen circulating in the bloodstream.

Estrogen receptors: The part of a cell, particularly sexual characteristic cells like breast cells, that allow the cell to recognize estrogen. Estrogen can be thought of as a key and the receptor as a lock, so estrogen opens the lock and allows the function to be performed, properly and naturally, or not.

Fibroadenoma: A non-cancerous lump commonly found in the breast(s), made up of fibrous tissue that can be as small as a pea or as large as a lemon. Fibroadenomas are generally found in teenagers and women in their early twenties, but they can occur at any age. In most cases, fibroadenomas do not need to be removed unless they are large, painful, or increasing in size. Usually they shrink on their own.

Folliculitis: Folliculitis of the breast is an inflammation of the hair follicles around the nipple area. A hair root becomes infected, which can be a mild infection or a chronic problem. Usually tiny red bumps appear. The bumps are often itchy and can become filled with pus.

Galactorrhea: A milky discharge from a woman's nipple other than breast milk. This can be caused by high levels of the hormone prolactin.

Gland: An organ in the body that releases a fluid that is used by the body at another location.

HER2: An aggressive type of cancer cell with hormone receptors.

Hereditary: Usually refers to a disease or characteristic that more than one family member or blood relative has. Eye color, height, and weight are some hereditary traits that can be inherited from family members.

Hormone: A chemical messenger that is released by an organ or gland and sent through the bloodstream to another part of the body.

Hormone imbalance: A condition that occurs when someone has either too much or too little of certain hormones.

LCIS: Lobular carcinoma in situ: Changes in the cells of the lobules or the milk-secreting ducts of the breast. LCIS is not visible on mammograms or MRIs. It is usually discovered when a sample of breast tissue is taken and examined under a microscope after a biopsy or when a breast lump is removed.

Mammary gland: A mammary gland is a body part or structure that is found inside a woman's breast. Mammary glands are shaped like lobes. These glands have an important function when a woman breastfeeds her baby because they work to secrete breast milk.

Menarche: The beginning of menstruation.

Menopause: The absence of menstrual periods for one year.

Menstruation: The monthly release of blood from a woman's uterus.

Metastasis: The spreading of cancer cells to another part of the body. Breast cancer cells frequently metastasize to the lungs, bone or liver.

Oncologist: A cancer specialist. These are often divided into subspecialties according to the type of cancer and the type of treatment.

Papillary mound: The nipple.

Perimenopause: The beginning of hormonal changes that signal the approach of menopause.

Prolactin: A hormone made by the pituitary gland that causes breast milk production.

Progesterone: A natural hormone made by the ovaries that sustains pregnancy, nurtures the fertilized egg and helps the body manufacture estrogen and testosterone.

Progestin: A synthetic substance meant to mimic progesterone.

Tanner Staging System: Also known as the sexual maturity rating, this five-stage system gauges a girl's transition through puberty.

Thelarche: The beginning of breast development as puberty approaches

Ultrasound: A method of imaging body tissue. Pictures produced using ultrasounds are very similar to x-ray photographs. However, when ultrasound is used, the images are produced using sound waves instead of x-rays. Ultrasound is a good way to examine breast lumps.

Yeast infection: An infection that is caused by the overgrowth of a fungus, which can cause a rash under the breasts, in the vagina or in other parts of the body.

BIOGRAPHIES

Dr. Ben, more formally known as Ben Johnson, *M.D., D.O., N.M.D.,* is a rare breed of physician who has degrees in conventional and complementary forms of medicine. His book learning and hands on experience are the foundation of the bridge he has built between several forms of medicine. He brings his expertise into focus with the highest good of the patient always in mind. In addition to treating patients, Dr. Ben has turned his focus on education through his work as cofounder of *The Healing Codes*™ and on his website, www.breastwisdombook.com. You're invited to visit the website for updates on material presented in this book and Dr. Ben's schedule.

Kathleen Barnes is the author of five natural health books and editor of several others. Her passion for natural health and sustainable living has its roots in the early days of the natural health movement. Kathleen has been part of the effort to raise public awareness of natural heath as an advocate and yoga teacher for more than 30 years. You can find more of her work at www.kathleenbarnes.com.